Dr. Miriam Stoppard

HRT

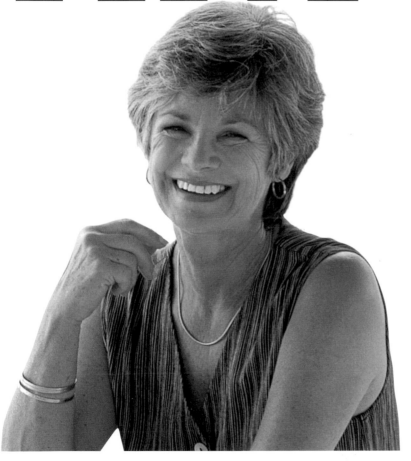

HEALTHCARE

DORLING KINDERSLEY
London • New York • Sydney • Moscow

Visit us on the World Wide Web at www.dk.com

A DORLING KINDERSLEY BOOK

Visit us on the World Wide Web at
www.dk.com

DESIGN & EDITORIAL   Mason Linklater

ART EDITOR   Lynne Brown
SENIOR MANAGING
EDITOR   Corinne Roberts

SENIOR ART EDITOR   Karen Ward
SENIOR EDITOR   Penny Warren

PRODUCTION   Sarah Coltman

First published in Great Britain in 1999
This revised edition published in Great Britain in
2003 by Dorling Kindersley Limited
80 Strand London WC2R 0RL

Copyright © 1999
Dorling Kindersley Limited, London
Text copyright © 1999 Dr. Miriam Stoppard

Some material in this publication was previously
published by Dorling Kindersley in *Menopause*
by Dr. Miriam Stoppard

A CIP catalogue record for this book is available
from the British Library

ISBN 0-7513-6981-0
Reproduced in Singapore by Colourscan
Printed in Slovakia by Tlaciarne BB s.r.o.

CONTENTS

INTRODUCTION

For many women, the menopause can be a psychological, emotional and intellectual turning point as well as a physical one, but it does not have to mean a decline. As your children leave home and you look forward to reducing your workload, you will have more time to yourself than ever before. This can be liberating and you can take the opportunity to reassess your lifestyle, your working patterns, decide what you want from the future and make some positive changes.

As the menopause approaches, the ovaries begin to fail and there is a sudden dip in our female sex hormones, oestrogen and progesterone, which causes the cessation of menstruation. About three-quarters of all women have some symptoms referable to the suddenness of oestrogen withdrawal, all of which can be treated. There is no need to slide on to the sidelines or to succumb to middle-aged spread if you don't want to. A good diet, combined with exercises to maintain strong, healthy bones, will enable you to keep your shape and self-confidence.

Symptoms of the menopause may be both long- and short-term. Short-term symptoms include hot flushes, night sweats and loss of libido, and some women can experience these for ten years or more. Long-term symptoms include the thinning and drying out of the vaginal and genital skin, and urinary troubles; these may all become permanent. Fortunately, these complaints are not dangerous and can be remedied by many therapies. However, some of the other consequences of the menopause are dangerous and are like bombs waiting to explode. These are osteoporosis or brittle bones, and one in four women who is admitted to hospital with a fractured thigh bone never leaves, so it is important that we are all protected from this disease. Oestrogens depress blood cholesterol and protect us from all forms of heart and vascular disease, and this includes heart attacks and strokes. In this respect, they are truly life-saving.

The positively good news is that hormone replacement therapy (HRT) can alleviate menopausal symptoms, and many different types are available, such as tablets, skin patches, creams, pessaries and implants. This means that nearly every woman can take HRT without suffering side-effects. With knowledge about how HRT affects your body, you can negotiate with your doctor on your own terms. In addition to medical help, there are many strategies that you can adopt to manage your treatment. There is a whole range of alternative therapies, from yoga to aromatherapy.

THE WHOLE PERSON

Any discussion of the menopause will run into controversy. Although we know that 98 percent of menopausal symptoms can be relieved by HRT, hormone replacement is by no means the only way to treat symptoms, which may be related to redundancy, changing family structure, a crisis of self-confidence, or a partner who is himself at one of life's crossroads. In any case, the menopause affects every organ of a woman's body, and any treatment must be viewed in the context of what is good for the whole; that involves diet, exercise, relaxation, yoga, vitamins, minerals and whatever change in your lifestyle you think would help. Each of the alternative therapies has its own champions.

Pills
This form of HRT relieves menopausal symptoms and also protects you against brittle bone disease.

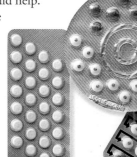

Far and away the two subjects that remain most hotly debated are, "is the menopause a hormone (oestrogen) deficiency condition?" and, following on from that, "should HRT be made available to any woman who wants to try it?" The first question is crucial because, if your answer is "yes", as mine is, then the inevitable conclusion is that treatment with HRT is justified. After all, no one disagrees with daily insulin injections for a person who has ceased to produce the hormone insulin.

Some medical experts claim that there is no hormone deficiency during the menopause because small amounts of oestrogen are manufactured in fat cells and during exercise. But these amounts are tiny compared to the amounts that we secrete when we are fertile, and when oestrogen falls below a certain level, symptoms such as hot flushes, and frequent, urgent urination can appear, and bone mass decreases. It's then a question of whether these symptoms should be treated. I believe that any symptom that is distressing deserves treating and, while other therapies may help, only HRT has a predictable success rate of 90 percent or above.

IS THE MENOPAUSE NATURAL?

We also face the argument that "the menopause is natural and should be left alone". It isn't natural. Even if it were, it shouldn't be dismissed as trivial, and by no means everything that is natural is good. The menopause is a mistake of nature. Women were never intended to forgo oestrogen. The human female wasn't meant to live beyond her fertile age. Up to the end of the 19th century the average woman didn't live long enough to experience the menopause. Simply because we are now able to prolong life 30 or 40 years beyond the menopause doesn't mean that women should be penalized with heart disease and osteoporosis (both natural consequences of living beyond 60)

when both of these conditions can be easily prevented with HRT. Prevention is always better than cure. Why ignore one of the most potent tools of preventive medicine because of prejudice and woolly thinking?

A big part of the "it's natural" argument is that the menopause is said to be part of the natural ageing process. It isn't. It is due to ovarian failure. Men suffer no comparable drop in their hormones and it is unjust to expect women to put up with sudden and almost complete withdrawal of their sex hormones.

At the time of the menopause there are profound hormonal changes that may lead to debilitating symptoms in the short-term and fatal diseases in the long-term. In every other area of medicine, doctors act to change malfunctions and correct mistakes of nature. It's simply inconsistent to exclude the menopause from this principle.

There still remains the controversy over who can take HRT. Alarming stories exist about HRT being the cause of breast cancer, uterine cancer and blood clots, and therefore dangerous in anyone who has a history of illness related to increased coagulability of the blood, such as heart attack or stroke. What we have to remember is that we all have a risk of most things, be it breast cancer, heart disease or pulmonary embolism. Recent US research has shown a small increase in cases of breast cancer in women taking certain types of HRT not available in the UK. But I believe that this very small additional risk, roughly equivalent to delaying your first baby till after 30 or drinking a glass of wine a day, must be weighed against the many benefits HRT confers, which include protection against osteoporosis and bowel cancer and possibly against Alzheimer's disease too. The link between HRT and uterine cancer was referable to the predominantly American habit of prescribing oestrogen without progestogen. Twenty years ago, research in Europe eradicated the possibility of uterine cancer by adding progestogen to the HRT regime. The US lags behind the rest of the world in adhering to this safe method of prescribing HRT and retains a prejudice against HRT.

WHEN NOT TO TAKE HRT

Largely because of regulations and possible litigation, drug companies still include long lists of contraindications to HRT on their pack inserts. These lists are outdated. Having performed a careful literature search, I have been unable to find an absolute ban on the use of HRT, since in the hands of an interested and sympathetic gynaecologist or doctor, there is always a way round the problem.

Even when facing the thorny question of previous breast cancer, the aim of HRT should be to alleviate menopausal symptoms while minimizing risks. A sensitive doctor will present the risk/benefit ratio of HRT to a woman – something doctors do every day with other medications – and help her to weigh up the pros and cons. The severity of a woman's symptoms and their impact on her life should be considered in relation to the potential risks of HRT. These risks can be vastly diminished if the doctor uses his or her imagination about the dose and method of taking HRT. For example, vaginal oestrogen in the form of a cream or a pessary can relieve vaginal and urinary symptoms, and restore sexual pleasure, yet, because the hormones are mainly confined to the pelvis, they will not affect the breasts. (Some oestrogen from creams or pessaries does pass into the bloodstream though, so care needs to be taken with the dosage and frequency of use.) In some women, hot flushes may be relieved by using the progestogenic drug, tibolone (see p. 49), which has no adverse effect on the breasts. Research is currently underway to evaluate the safety of adding a small daily dose of the drug tamoxifen to HRT for women who have had breast cancer. Tamoxifen is given to premenopausal women to treat breast cancer. There are no longer any grounds for a doctor to deny a woman HRT or to refuse to discuss it with her. Not all women need oestrogen, but I firmly believe that all women should have the choice. Indeed, I would go further: all women have the right to a four-month trial of HRT. After all, you have nothing to lose (you won't incur any risk with such short-term dosage) and everything to gain. In four months you will know if the quality of your life has improved.

We have not only made it possible for all women to take HRT if they want to, but we have defined a group of women who need HRT – women who would experience a measurable benefit in terms of life expectancy. Anyone who has taken steroids or has a family history of bowel cancer can be protected from conditions like osteoporosis and bowel cancer by taking HRT. If you are among them, you should be demanding HRT from your doctor.

EXPLAINING THE MENOPAUSE

As the supply of eggs in a woman's ovaries dwindles, the two hormones, oestrogen and progesterone, fluctuate and then begin to decline. This produces the hallmark of midlife – the end of menstrual periods – but it also has manifold effects on the rest of the body. Menopausal symptoms are felt largely because of the suddenness of oestrogen withdrawal; if this deficiency is counteracted with HRT, good diet and proper exercise, bones will remain strong, hair and skin will stay healthy and you will keep your shape, and positive attitudes to life.

*To understand the difference
between "menopause" and
"climacteric", it may help to
think of the menopause as
being the counterpart of the
menarche, which was the
time when your periods
started. The climacteric can
be compared with the years
of adolescence or puberty
when your ovaries began
functioning and maturing.
The following points clarify
the differences between the
menopause and climacteric.*

Menopause …
• *is comparable to menarche.*

• *is a single biological event.*

• *means cessation of periods.*

• *occurs usually between the
ages of 48 and 52.*

Climacteric …
• *is comparable to puberty.*

• *involves a series of hormonal
changes.*

• *is a transitional phase when
ovarian function and hormone
production decline.*

• *usually spans the ages of
40–60.*

WHAT HAPPENS TO YOUR BODY

The end of fertile life doesn't have to imply new restrictions and physical decline; our options can increase rather than decrease. Try to remember the following positive statements:

• Being well informed and prepared for the menopause will help you deal effectively with symptoms.

• You deserve sympathy and understanding from your partner and family as much as you did at any other time of your life.

• The speed of ageing does not suddenly accelerate after the menopause.

• The menopause is not an unmentionable subject. If you experience menopausal symptoms, talk about them. The more open you are about it, the more you will help to break down taboos.

• You have the right to take control of this stage of your life, as much as any other stage. If you don't want to rely on doctors or medicines, you don't have to. There are plenty of relaxation and meditation techniques, as well as complementary and dietary approaches that can help you deal with symptoms effectively and successfully.

• There is no reason why the menopause should be a time of sexual decline. You can take steps to maintain and even improve the quality of your sex life even though there is less oestrogen in your body.

• There's no time like the present for developing a new hobby or project. You can even take up a second career.

• You should embark on financial planning for retirement as early as possible, to take advantage of what are potentially your most creative years. Financial planning is helpful if you have to simplify your life as you grow older.

• Femininity does not have to equal fertility. The menopause is not the beginning of the end; it's the beginning of the rest of your life.

THE MENOPAUSE TIMETABLE

To understand the changes that happen to us during the menopause, it is necessary to understand the terminology that doctors and others use (see left). Most of the time we use the word "menopause" incorrectly. Strictly speaking, the menopause means the end of menstruation, and could hypothetically be a single moment in time. The word "climacteric" more accurately describes the ongoing changes and symptoms, since it refers to a phase or transition period that may last 15–20 years. During this phase, ovarian function and hormonal production decline, and the body adjusts itself to these changes. The word climacteric comes from a Greek word that, literally translated, means "rung of a ladder".

THE CLIMACTERIC

This can be divided into three stages: the premenopause, perimenopause and postmenopause. The menopause is a point in time that signals the end of the premenopause and the beginning of the postmenopause.

Premenopause This refers to the years when your menstrual cycle is regular; in other words, most of your fertile, reproductive life. However, "premenopause" is also sometimes used to refer to the early years of the climacteric, after the age of 40, when menstrual periods may become irregular or heavy. If your doctor ever tells you that you are premenopausal, you should ask for a precise definition of what he or she means.

Perimenopause This is the stage lasting several years on either side of your last menstrual period. This means that the perimenopause is, in part, a retrospective diagnosis, since it's only when your periods cease that you can measure backwards two years in time to know when your perimenopause began. Vague symptoms that you may not have connected in your own mind can become significant when viewed as part of the perimenopause. It's during this time that you notice most physical changes, when your periods may become irregular and when hot flushes or night sweats may start.

Menopause This has a very precise meaning – the menopause is your final menstrual period. This is another date that can be identified only retrospectively, when you have not had a menstrual bleed for 12 months. In other words, it is impossible for a woman to know the exact moment in time that she is experiencing the menopause.

CAN I PREDICT MY LAST PERIOD?

Most women anticipate that they will experience their last menstrual period around 50, although the average age for the menopause in the UK is 51 years of age.

About a third of all women stop menstruating before their 45th birthday, but this is not necessarily a sign of any abnormality. At the other end of the scale, many women go on menstruating into their early 50s, and a few continue into their mid-50s. Studies done in the United States show that 90 percent of women experience a natural menopause by the age of 54, and 100 percent of women have stopped menstruating by the age of 58.

Although there is no way in which you can predict exactly when your menopause will occur, research has shown that there are several factors that may influence its timing. It is thought that the age you begin to menstruate may affect the age that you experience the menopause, but no studies have yet proved this. It is possible that the age at which your mother experienced the menopause will have some bearing on when you stop menstruating, but again this relationship has not been scientifically proven.

Two factors that definitely do not influence the time of your menopause are whether or not you took the oral contraceptive pill, or your age when you had your first and last child.

FAT BEFORE THE MENOPAUSE

Throughout fertile life, the hormones oestrogen and progesterone are responsible for maintaining the female shape, with its narrow waist and rounded hips. We now know that these proportions are more than simply an expression of the female gender. They have a great significance for both health and longevity.

The narrow waist and rounded hips pattern of fat distribution is closely related to coronary health. The usual ratio of the waist to hip measurement is less than one and this is associated with a low risk of a heart attack. If your waist to hip ratio creeps above 0.8, you are much more at risk (see p. 31).

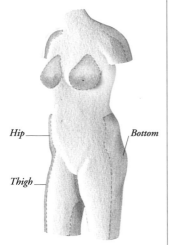

Hip ——

—— Bottom

Thigh ——

Distribution of fat
During the fertile years, fat (coloured yellow) tends to accumulate on the hips, bottom and upper thighs.

Postmenopause This overlaps with the end of the perimenopausal stage and will extend into the years that follow your last menstrual period right up until the end of your life.

MIDLIFE MENSTRUAL CHANGES

I'd like to begin by saying what does not happen during the menopause – or what *need* not happen at this time. Myths abound and they are rarely contradicted because, as Gail Sheehy explained in her book *The Silent Passage*, the menopause is not often talked about. The first myth I'd like to explode is that the menopause is a disease. Like pregnancy, which has also become "medicalized" in Western culture, the menopause should be monitored carefully so that problems are avoided, abnormalities are corrected and complications are treated, but in no way is it a disease. Nor is the menopause a psychological crisis. It may be a change, but we cope with a series of changes in our lives without drama. And looking back, we would regard many changes as positive, particularly if they free us to focus on priorities. The menopause does not usher in old age – it is part of a continual life cycle. Postmenopausal women don't lose their femininity, nor do they stop being attractive. Far from it. As we get older we take on fresh allure and sex appeal, based on wisdom and confidence.

It is well known that the menopause can very occasionally occur in women in their teens and early twenties, but the average age in the Western world is 51 years. The climacteric – the interval between the beginning and the end of menopausal symptoms – can span seven or more years. During this time your menstrual cycle will become increasingly irregular and, ultimately, menstruation ceases completely and the menopause occurs.

Menstrual changes vary from woman to woman. Some women experience a shorter cycle – menstruation every 20 or so days is not uncommon; others find themselves menstruating less frequently, perhaps only once every six months. The flow pattern may also change; a woman may go on bleeding regularly but notice that the number of days of menstrual flow are fewer, or that the flow itself is diminished. On the other hand, flow may increase. You could have a shorter cycle with heavier bleeding, or fewer cycles with many days of very light flow. However, less bleeding less often is the commonest pattern.

Ninety percent of women who don't menstruate for six months will not menstruate again. But some women may have intervals of no periods and then irregular periods for quite a number of years. It is important to understand that there is no fixed pattern of change.

FALLING HORMONE LEVELS

If you have a history of regular menstruation, your oestrogen and progesterone levels will have been changing daily in a predictable and orderly rhythm. As you become menopausal, your menstrual cycle is likely to change, reflecting the major upheavals in hormone secretion in your body. Oestrogen levels in the first two weeks of the cycle get lower and lower; this is because fewer egg follicles, which secrete oestrogen, are stimulated to grow. In addition, ovulation becomes less likely since the supply of eggs is running out. If ovulation does occur, conception is less likely, since the quality of the eggs released is more likely to be substandard.

Without ovulation there is no corpus luteum to produce progesterone (corpus luteum is the name given to an egg follicle after its release into the Fallopian tube). As a consequence, oestrogen stimulates the growth of the uterine lining in the first half of the month, which becomes unopposed by progesterone in the second half. Without progesterone the endometrium becomes thicker and thicker, until finally it breaks down naturally, resulting in heavy and prolonged bleeding.

From the age of about 35 the menstrual cycle becomes less consistent, and in the late 30s a woman may begin not to ovulate in every menstrual cycle. Without eggs, oestrogen and progesterone are not secreted, and the symptoms of the menopause begin to appear (see pp. 24–34). When oestrogen levels fall too low to stimulate the growth of the uterine lining, menstruation ceases.

With the decline of oestrogen and progesterone production, the hypothalamus and pituitary gland secrete larger and larger quantities of follicle-stimulating hormone (FSH) and luteinizing hormone (LH) to try to stimulate ovulation. The ovary, however, cannot respond consistently, despite the high hormone levels, and

FAT AFTER THE MENOPAUSE

After the menopause, when levels of the hormones oestrogen and progesterone are low or absent, one of the first things that a woman may notice is a thickening of the waist and the appearance of "middle-age spread".

You may also notice abdominal swelling because of increased fat on the front of your abdomen. Your shape comes to resemble a more masculine outline, and your risk of having a heart attack increases in relation to this increased fat distribution.

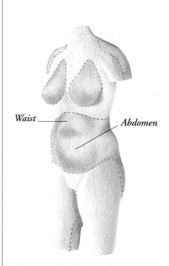

Waist ———

——— Abdomen

Changes in body shape
When a woman is no longer fertile, fat (coloured yellow) is concentrated around the waist and abdomen.

THE NORMAL MENSTRUAL CYCLE

Oestrogen is secreted by developing egg follicles in the ovary. The level of oestrogen rises and peaks in the first half of the menstrual cycle.

This is followed by ovulation, and the egg follicle that is left behind changes into a structure called a corpus luteum. This produces progesterone and smaller amounts of oestrogen. Bleeding occurs when oestrogen and progesterone levels drop.

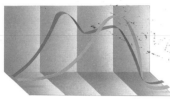

DAY 1   7   14   21   28

KEY   OESTROGEN

           PROGESTERONE

           MENSTRUATION

women may experience normal menstrual cycles interspersed by cycles of troublesome oestrogen deficiency. High levels of FSH and LH alone can disturb many aspects of a woman's metabolism, including brain chemistry, mood, thyroid function, bone integrity, fat metabolism and blood sugar levels.

A HORMONE DEFICIENCY STATE?

Some doctors regard the menopause as natural, and interference with it as unnatural and unnecessary. I disagree. While I believe that the menopause is a normal stage in the development of a woman's life, I also believe that it is a true hormone deficiency state. Just as a deficiency of the hormone insulin gives rise to diabetes, lack of oestrogen and progesterone can give rise to osteoporosis, heart disease and stroke. There is no question as to whether or not the symptoms of diabetes should be treated, and I think women have the right to treatment for menopausal symptoms.

Women have two major oestrogens – oestradiol and its breakdown product, oestrone. The levels of both start to decline even before there are any symptoms of the menopause. As a result, the blood level of FSH (follicle-stimulating hormone) starts to rise, and a blood test that shows this heralds the menopause. Women at any menopausal stage are eligible for hormone replacement therapy (HRT, see pp. 43–60). At the very least, they should be given hormone supplements to smooth out the dramatic fall-off of female sex hormones, and serious consideration must also be given to long-term hormone supplements, which can help to stave off life-threatening diseases, for example osteoporosis, commonly called "brittle bone disease" (see pp. 70–76).

Every organ in a woman's body is, in some way, affected by oestrogen and progesterone. There are at least 400 actions of oestrogen at a cellular level alone. Practically every important body tissue contains oestrogen receptors that keep the body normal and stimulate its function. When the secretion of oestrogen and progesterone varies, the health and well-being of our organs reflects these changes. For example, in each premenstrual week, the decline in hormones can result in mood changes and fluid retention. If your menstrual cycle is roughly lunar (28 days long), you will experience relative oestrogen and progesterone deficiency 13 times a year. This is equivalent to a tiny menopause each month and probably explains why women have premenstrual tension.

Normally, we are largely unaware of bodily changes related to fluctuating hormone levels and we think about them only when our health is affected and symptoms such as muscle fatigue, bone pain and joint stiffness appear. As part of our female inheritance, we grow up with – and take for granted – a variety of symptoms that are due to fluctuating hormone levels.

During the normal menstrual cycle, oestradiol is the major oestrogen and it is synthesized by the developing follicle in the ovary. After the menopause, oestrone takes over as the major oestrogen. Rather than being produced in the ovaries, oestrone is made by a secondary process in fat cells and muscles; it is synthesized from the male sex hormone androstenedione, which continues to be secreted by the postmenopausal ovaries and the adrenal glands. Because oestrone is not produced cyclically after the menopause, the rate of its formation does not fluctuate in the way that oestradiol did premenopausally. Oestrone is also biologically much less active than oestradiol, and this can manifest itself as a relative excess of male hormones in the body. This means that our overall hormonal profile begins to move nearer to that of men. The most visible signs of this shift are the appearance of facial hair, male-pattern baldness and the tendency to put on weight around the waist and the abdomen (in the premenopausal years fat is laid down on the hips rather than on the waist). However, the most dangerous change is one that is invisible: cardiovascular health deteriorates, bringing the rate of female heart disease into line with the rate of male heart disease. Supplementing your natural oestrogen with HRT may lessen the chances of these changes occurring.

HOW THE BODY CHANGES

Some women find the experience of the menopause particularly disconcerting because they feel that their bodies are changing, even letting them down, and they really can't understand why or how. You will be better prepared to cope with the following changes if you have an understanding of why they are taking place and what you can do to prevent them.

HORMONES DURING THE MENOPAUSE

Until the menopause, the hormones oestrogen and progesterone are produced in approximately a 28-day cycle (see column, left). When the supply of eggs runs out in midlife, hormone production becomes erratic.

Oestrogen is produced by eggs in the ovary, but sometimes no single maturing egg becomes dominant, and so ovulation does not occur. This means that progesterone is not secreted in every cycle, and a menstrual bleed may not occur in every cycle. Since hormone levels can fluctuate dramatically at this time, women may experience menopausal symptoms.

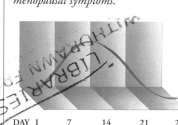

DAY 1   7   14   21   28

KEY   ∿   OESTROGEN

      ▦   MENSTRUATION

POST-MENOPAUSAL HORMONES

Oestrogen is present in small amounts after ovulation and menstruation have ceased; it is mainly converted by the fat cells from the male sex hormone androstenedione.

Because ovulation no longer takes place, there is no corpus luteum, and progesterone is absent. Unless you are taking HRT, any bleeding that you experience after the menopause should be considered abnormal.

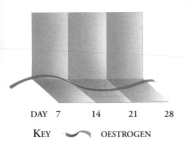

DAY   7   14   21   28

KEY ⟿ OESTROGEN

UROGENITAL TISSUE

The cells of the urethra and the vagina contain oestrogen receptors that bind with oestrogen, keeping the tissues healthy. When oestrogen levels start to fall at the menopause, the results include a decrease in blood supply to the tissues and a lowering of cellular starch. The latter leads to a change in the acidity of the vagina so that it becomes a more alkaline environment. This encourages vaginal soreness, itching and infections. Similar cellular changes are seen in the lining of the urethra, giving rise to urgent, frequent or uncomfortable urination. Applying oestrogen cream to the area may reverse these changes and relieve symptoms. Urogenital problems will also respond to other forms of HRT.

UTERUS

This is a smooth muscle with an inner lining, known as the endometrium, which contains glands and blood vessels. The endometrium builds up and breaks down each month throughout a woman's fertile life, unless she is pregnant. In about half of all menopausal women the endometrium begins to thin out, becoming what is called atrophic (in this context, atrophic simply means "thinned out"). The endometrial thickness depends on how much oestrogen is present in a woman's body, whether manufactured by conversion from adrenal androgens (male sex hormones) or introduced to the body in the form of HRT.

FALLOPIAN TUBES

During the fertile years, waves of contraction pass down the Fallopian tubes. Such movements help to transport your ovum to the cavity of the uterus, and sperm towards the waiting egg. After the menopause, when oestrogen levels decline, the internal cellular structure of the tubes begins to regress and the tubes become immobile. Fortunately, these internal changes have no detrimental effect on your general well-being and fitness.

OVARIES

As women approach the menopause, the declining number of eggs in the ovaries means that ovulation will not necessarily take place in every 28-day cycle. This in turn results in the secretion of oestrogen becoming erratic and women may experience various menopausal symptoms, such as hot flushes and night sweats. After the menopause, the egg follicles in the ovary no longer grow and mature each month. Ovulation does not occur, and this means that there is no ruptured egg follicle (corpus luteum, see column p. 14), and therefore little progesterone is produced.

The outer shell of the ovary, which produced oestrogen and progesterone during your fertile life, becomes thinner and wrinkled, and the entire ovary shrinks. However, during the postmenopause, the inner part of the ovary continues actively to secrete hormones, principally the male hormones, androstenedione and testosterone. The latter is important in keeping up your energy and enthusiasm for life. Unfortunately, it also promotes changes in your fat metabolism that increase your risk of suffering from life-threatening conditions such as heart disease and stroke (see pp. 31–33). Androstenedione is converted in small quantities to the weak female hormone, oestrone (a form of oestrogen), which helps to maintain the health of the pelvic organs, the skin, the hair and the vagina. If you have your ovaries surgically removed, you lose a significant source of postmenopausal oestrogen and it is important to take HRT.

VAGINA

When oestrogen levels drop, the vagina begins to atrophy (this simply means that it becomes thin and dry). While not all women are affected, the activity of the glands in the vagina does begin to wane for many women as they get older. Healthy mucus is no longer secreted to keep the vagina lubricated, and it becomes more prone to infection and abrasions, which can lead to pain and bleeding during intercourse. Such vaginal discomfort is a primary reason for loss of sex drive in postmenopausal women, and you may find that you need to use a lubricant to enable penetration. If you go to your doctor, he or she may prescribe oestrogen pessaries or cream, which will restore the vaginal lining to its premenopausal state. Research shows that women who remain sexually active after the menopause suffer less from vaginal atrophy than women who do not masturbate or who do not have sexual intercourse.

PELVIC FLOOR

The muscles of the pelvic floor give support to all the pelvic organs, including the rectum, bladder and uterus.

Without adequate levels of oestrogen, this support structure loses its tension, elasticity and strength during and after the menopause. This means that pelvic organs, particularly the uterus, are no longer well supported by the pelvic floor muscles and are inclined to sag or prolapse. The vagina may also be affected, resulting in a loss of sensation during sexual intercourse. Doing pelvic floor exercises, called Kegel exercises, can combat this (see Exercise and Sex, p. 26).

When the vaginal walls are thin and stretched, the rectum, bladder and urethra can prolapse down through the front or back of the vagina (see pp. 88–89). This may be avoided if HRT is taken to maintain the strength and elasticity of the pelvic support structure (unless prolapse is due to damage during childbirth). Local HRT, such as oestrogen cream or gel, will keep the pelvic organs healthy while avoiding most side-effects.

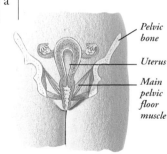

Pelvic bone

Uterus

Main pelvic floor muscle

HAIR

The growth and rest cycle, and the health of each hair, are maintained by oestrogen receptors in the hair follicles. When oestrogen levels are low, hair growth is disturbed.

For this reason, hair growth patterns change at the time of the menopause and beyond. You may notice that your hair loses its body and thickness, and becomes thinner, finer and more difficult to style. This must be distinguished from alopecia, where patches of total hair loss occur, and from male pattern baldness, which may occur in women who have a substantial excess of androgens (male sex hormones). The average age of hormonally related hair loss is about 60. No cure is known at present.

The other major change in hair growth is hirsutism – the growth of excess body hair. Unfortunately, facial hirsutism usually gets worse with age. If you are suffering from facial hirsutism, your doctor must identify the cause before any attempt at treatment is made.

VULVA AND PERINEUM

All structures of the vulva and perineum (the area between the vagina and anus) become less plump at the menopause. The labia minora and majora (vaginal lips) become thin and flat, the urethral opening becomes slack and wider, and the skin of the perineum becomes thinner and dryer. All of these changes can lead to itchiness and, in the extreme form, a condition called pruritus vulvae (see pp. 86–87). The changes can also lead to infections, and the area may be slow to heal. The use of oestrogen cream can completely reverse these changes, so that itchiness vanishes and healing occurs more rapidly.

BREASTS

As we get older the breasts tend to sag and flatten – the larger the breasts, the flatter they may become. With the menopause there is a reduction of oestrogen stimulation on all tissues in the body, including the breast tissues, and as a result, they lose their earlier fullness. There is also a reduction in the glandular tissue of the breast and an increase in fat cells. Women who take HRT will find that breast fullness is restored to a large degree and this will remain for as long as hormones are taken. Breast cancer is a risk after the menopause, and the later the menopause, the higher the risk. If you have breast cancer you should seek advice from a doctor or gynaecologist about HRT.

Some women suffer from breast tenderness or breast pain, known as mastalgia, at the time of the menopause. Mastalgia is no reason not to take HRT; in fact HRT often brings considerable relief.

ABDOMEN

If you exercise regularly, you should not experience any sudden changes in the size and shape of your abdomen. However, if you stop having periods and notice that your abdomen suddenly increases in size, you should consult your doctor, because a sudden enlargement of the abdomen is sometimes the only noticeable sign of an ovarian tumour (see p. 79).

Alternatively, if you feel bloated or distended and your waist size has grown, you may be eating a diet that is too low in fibre, or taking insufficient exercise. If you don't do much exercise, you will experience a gradual loss of abdominal wall tone. You will find that you simply cannot pull in your tummy the way you used to be able to. Healthy abdominal muscles support the internal organs. Regular muscle exercise makes a huge difference not only to the shape of your abdomen, but also to your self-image – and you're never too old to start a fitness programme. Wearing a girdle will actually promote the development of lazy musculature, leading to an increase in abdominal bulging.

CONNECTIVE TISSUE

The body consists of a skeleton, muscles and organs, surrounded by skin and supported by a scaffolding of connective tissue, such as that found in gristle. The major component of connective tissue is collagen, which is kept healthy by oestrogen. After the menopause the body loses collagen from everywhere, and connective tissue becomes weak. Bones become brittle, muscles become weaker and joints become stiffer. Skin becomes thinner and wrinkles. The vagina thins, causing pain on sexual intercourse and the symptoms of cystitis appear (see pp. 85–86). All of this is due to the disintegration of collagen contingent on low oestrogen levels.

BONES

Despite its solid appearance, bone is actually porous and becomes more porous with age. There are two types of cells that actively influence bone health. The cells known as osteoblasts are responsible for building up bone, and those known as osteoclasts are responsible for the removal or resorption of bone. At the time of the menopause the activity of the osteoclasts becomes greater than that of the osteoblasts. In other words, more bone is removed than is created, and bone mass and density are lost. The decline of oestrogen is responsible for this.

While a woman is still menstruating, the presence of oestrogen in her body allows her to fully utilize other hormones, such as calcitonin and parathyroid, and vitamins, such as vitamin D, all of which influence bone health. Parathyroid hormone and calcitonin both keep the amount of calcium in the body at a constant level (in particular, parathyroid hormone prevents too much calcium from being lost from the urine by acting on the

SKIN

Decline of oestrogen during the menopause is one of the things that accelerates skin ageing, and you should really take special care of your skin after the age of 40. As you get older, the following skin changes occur:

- *Its ability to spring back into shape is lost.*

- *It is less easily compressed and loses its mobility.*

- *Water-filled cells lose their turgidity (plumpness).*

- *There is a decrease in total skin collagen, which is one of the main supporting proteins in your skin. The structure of the skin starts to collapse and wrinkles appear. Ultraviolet (UV) light is largely responsible for the break-up of collagen fibres in the skin.*

- *There is a continual loss of cells called melanocytes, which manufacture the pigment melanin. Melanin causes your skin to become tanned in the sun, so as you grow older its loss means that you are more prone to sunburn, and in turn to collagen destruction and skin cancer. It is crucial that you guard your skin from the damaging rays of the sun. Use high-protection sunscreens with an SPF factor of at least 20, wear a hat to shield your face and, when possible, limit your exposure to the sun.*

CALCIUM METABOLISM

This is specifically linked to bone health, which declines with the menopause.

Oestrogen plays an important role in keeping blood calcium levels normal by aiding the absorption of calcium from food. It also promotes absorption of calcium from the blood into the bone, assisting the renewal and repair activity of osteoblasts (see Bones, p. 19). When oestrogen levels in the body fall, calcium absorption is less efficient and uptake of calcium into the bone slows down so that the bones may become brittle.

kidneys and by increasing calcium absorption from food). Insufficient oestrogen in a woman's body during and after the menopause means that calcium is lost from the body, making bones weaker and prone to brittleness (see Osteoporosis, pp. 70–76).

Although hip fractures are common in women with osteoporosis, they tend to affect older women in their 70s. Women who are recently postmenopausal and have osteoporosis are more likely to suffer from Colles' fracture (wrist fracture), or vertebral fracture. Women who are diagnosed as being at risk of osteoporosis can prevent their bones from deteriorating by taking HRT.

MUSCLES AND JOINTS

With advancing age and a decline in oestrogen and progesterone production, the muscular system loses its strength, bulk and stamina. The average elderly person has little muscle mass left and is at risk from a variety of problems. Weak muscles mean that many elderly people have poor coordination.

As collagen everywhere disintegrates at the time of the menopause, joints may become stiff and painful, and this is particularly noticeable on waking. Some studies have shown that two out of three women attending clinics for menopausal symptoms experience some joint discomfort or pain with limitation of movement. HRT can virtually eliminate these symptoms and regular exercise will ensure that joints stay mobile.

HEART AND BLOOD VESSELS

The exact effect the menopause has on the heart and blood vessels is not fully understood. What is known is that, irrespective of age, women with functioning ovaries are less prone to heart disease than women who have gone through the menopause either naturally or after surgical removal of the ovaries, such as by hysterectomy (see pp. 80–82). For example, women who experience a surgically induced menopause before the age of 35 have a two to seven times greater risk of a heart attack than pre-menopausal women with intact ovaries.

In the United States, close to half a million women a year die of a cardiovascular disease, and nearly all of them are postmenopausal. This figure is eight times higher than the combined death rate for all cancers of the reproductive system. Until oestrogen declines at the menopause, cardiovascular disease is almost never a cause of death in women.

Each year over one million postmenopausal American women experience a malfunction of the cardiovascular system. The heart may not pump adequately, the blood vessels may tear and form scar tissue, or dangerous fats travelling in the blood may clog and narrow the arteries; all of these affect blood circulation and compromise the pumping capacity of the heart, which can be fatal.

Cholesterol levels normally increase in women as they grow older. However, the levels increase at an even faster rate in women who have had their ovaries removed. Loss of ovarian function leads to an increase in the dangerous low-density type of cholesterol (LDL), and a reduction in the cardioprotective high-density cholesterol (HDL). These changes lead to heart disease, but may be controlled in women taking HRT. Oestrogen receptors have been found in the muscle layer of arteries; loss of oestrogen causes these muscles to tighten, which constricts the blood vessels and increases blood pressure. Reduction of blood pressure can occur within a few weeks of starting HRT.

EMOTIONS AND BEHAVIOUR

There are many sites in the brain where oestrogen receptors are found in high concentration. Oestradiol, our most active oestrogen, has at least 50 actions in the brain alone. Oestrogen receptors control function in the part of the brain, the hippocampus, that is responsible for memory, and this may explain why some women experience forgetfulness and memory loss before the other symptoms of the menopause.

Research into the effects of oestrogen on receptors in the brain is very revealing and provides great insight into the intellectual and emotional changes that menopausal women experience. The hippocampus is a part of the brain that oversees a complex system of information storage. Even during the menstrual cycle, its ability to store data fluctuates noticeably. Oestrogen controls cognitive functions such as conceptual thinking and perceptions, and qualities like having a flexible attitude to change. During the menopause these functions and qualities may become impaired. Low oestrogen levels

HOT FLUSHES AND NIGHT SWEATS

Oestrogen is responsible for control of body temperature. Without it, our "thermostat" fails, and we sweat profusely at normal temperatures.

For two-thirds of all women, hot flushes and night sweats start well before their last menstrual period. They tend to become worse in frequency and duration at the time of the menopause, and continue to occur, with occasional trouble-free months, for about the next five years. When you first begin to experience hot flushes they are usually infrequent and are on the face and neck only. Once they start, they tend to get worse before they get better.

Why does a hot flush come when it does, and what causes it? The reasons are complex, but the onset of a flush may correspond with an increase in the level of the pituitary hormone, luteinizing hormone (LH). Significant changes in levels of LH secretion are common as the menopause approaches (see p. 13) and appear to be a response to the shrinking of the ovaries and decreased oestrogen secretion.

Other internal secretions also surge during a hot flush. For example, there is a significant rise in the blood level of some of the adrenal hormones. Hot flushes and night sweats often cause insomnia (wakefulness) and a reduction in rapid eye movement (dream) sleep so that sleep is not as refreshing, contributing to fatigue.

BRAIN CONTROL OF MOVEMENT

Oestrogen appears to increase cellular metabolism in the brain even where there are no specific oestrogen receptors. This "tonic" effect is very apparent in the areas of the brain controlling our ability to make fine movements.

The cerebellum is the area of the brain that controls balance and coordination. Research has shown that taking oestrogen can bring about a threefold increase in cerebellar function within three minutes, which lasts for nine hours.

All kinds of muscular activities are improved by oestrogen stimulation, including manual dexterity. Without oestrogen, our ability to perform intricate movements, such as are needed to play the violin or guitar, for example, may be impaired.

The olive is the area of the brain that acts as a timing device, synchronizing movements to actions. For example, without correctly timed responses, we can trip over a kerb. The olive helps by sending out rhythmic electrical discharges that tell the cerebellum when to move muscles so that our movements are synchronized. After taking oestrogen, synchronicity of muscle movement improves markedly, and progesterone enhances the effect of the oestrogen. Studies also show that the olive is 30 percent more sensitive to errors when oestrogen levels are high.

affect our ability to learn new facts and skills, for example, and our ability to recall recently read material. HRT improves these skills. HRT also has a general "tonic" effect on the brain and so is thought to delay the onset of Alzheimer's disease.

Perhaps the most important finding is that oestrogen prevents anxiety, which may explain why anxiety is such a dominant symptom of the menopause. Some of the effects of oestrogen are as therapeutic as those of tranquillizers, and in a way, menopausal women are suffering from "natural tranquillizer withdrawal". Oestrogen has a wide-ranging role in combating anxiety, tension and depression, even encompassing the ability to adjust smoothly from light to darkness, finding a way through a strange environment, interacting with a stranger and taking criticism.

In contrast, progesterone receptors in the brain can bring on negative moods. In one study, women reported depression occurring within hours of taking progestogen (a synthetic form of progesterone). Progesterone receptors may account for the black moods that some women suffer during the days when progestogen is part of their HRT regime (see p. 57), and during the week before menstruation.

The amygdala is a centre in the brain responsible for psychological well-being and sexuality, and it contains hundreds of oestrogen receptors that maintain its ability to respond to stimuli. Loss of oestrogen reduces the amygdala's excitability, resulting in a lowered sense of well-being and diminished sex drive. Women taking HRT experience increased arousal and more sexual fantasies than previously.

HOW YOU CAN MANAGE YOUR MENOPAUSE

The list of symptoms associated with the menopause is long, and all are connected to a drop in oestrogen levels. Fortunately, no woman experiences the whole range of symptoms; you will probably have only a few and many women have none. The physical effects of the menopause are so diverse, it is sometimes hard to connect them to a single cause. Some classic symptoms, such as hot flushes and mood swings, are readily associated with the menopause; others, like back pain, often seem incidental.

The following simple measures can relieve symptoms.

• *Record your flushes; try to avoid recurrence of situations that act as a trigger.*

• *Don't wear synthetic fabrics, and avoid clothes with high necks and long sleeves.*

• *Discover ways of cooling down: keep a thermos flask of iced water near you, take a cold shower, or use a fan.*

• *Give up smoking.*

MEDICAL TREATMENT

Hormone replacement therapy (HRT, see pp. 43–60) has a 98 percent success rate at relieving hot flushes and night sweats.

Clonidine, propranolol (drugs for the treatment of high blood pressure) and sedative drugs may also be helpful. Ask your doctor for advice.

THE RANGE OF SYMPTOMS

The list described here is long simply because it's helpful to know the array of disparate symptoms, especially if you need to discuss your treatment with a doctor.

HOT FLUSHES AND NIGHT SWEATS

A night sweat is the night-time equivalent of a hot flush; both of these are experienced by more than 85 percent of menopausal women, although their frequency and severity varies greatly from woman to woman. During a hot flush or night sweat, a woman can perspire so profusely that perspiration runs down her face, neck and back; her body temperature will rise, her heart will beat faster and she may also experience palpitations. Very occasionally, a woman may faint during a hot flush, but this is rare.

Even though a hot flush and night sweat may feel most severe in the head, face and neck, the rise in temperature occurs throughout the body. Even the finger and toe temperatures rise sharply at the beginning of a flush.

The discomfort from a hot flush or night sweat is unique – it's not the same as simply being overheated. In one study, investigators tried to induce hot flushes in menopausal women using hot water bottles and blankets. They found that applying external heat does not produce the same dramatic changes in heart rate and blood pressure that a menopausal flush does. However, night sweats can be aggravated by hot weather.

COMPLEMENTARY THERAPY

The products that herbalists and homeopaths most often suggest for hot flushes and night sweats are pulsatilla, lachesis, goldenseal, wild yam root, black cohosh, sage, soya beans, *fo-ti-tieng* and *dong quai*. Most healthfood shops and pharmacies that sell natural products stock all of them; or consult a qualified herbalist or homeopath. Agnus castus is an excellent herb for many menopausal symptoms including hot flushes and night sweats.

Relaxation can be particularly therapeutic because it calms the mind and body, which in turn normalizes body chemistry and makes the skin sweat less. Meditation can be useful too. It slows down your metabolism, and it can slow down your brain waves from the fast beta waves that are characteristic of the working day to a slower alpha or theta wave, the wave pattern that occurs just before sleeping; if you can achieve a meditative state it can be as restful as sleep. Beginners' yoga, with its simple postures and deep breathing techniques, can also have a calming effect.

DIET AND EXERCISE

Limit foods and drinks that trigger hot flushes and night sweats. These include dishes that are sugary, salty or spicy, chocolate, alcohol, coffee, tea and cola drinks. Hot soups and drinks or large meals can also trigger a night sweat or hot flush. Eat plenty of citrus fruits, such as oranges and grapefruit; these contain bioflavonoids, which have a weak oestrogenic effect on the body.

Take regular physical exercise; women who exercise tend to have fewer hot flushes and night sweats than those who don't. Exercise vastly improves the circulation, and it can make your body more tolerant of temperature extremes and better able to cool down quickly. Exercise also helps to increase the amount of oestrogen and endorphins (chemicals with a feel-good effect) circulating in the blood. The more oestrogen that you have, the less chance there is of your having a hot flush or night sweat.

VAGINAL AND URINARY PROBLEMS

Urogenital problems are very common during the menopause, yet only four in ten women consult their doctor about them. Anatomically, the vagina and the lower urinary tract lie very close, separated by just a few layers of cells. They both respond to a lack of oestrogen by becoming thin and dry.

Urinary symptoms typically include discomfort when passing urine, and the desire to urinate frequently and urgently, even if there is very little urine in the bladder. There may also be some dribbling because the sphincter muscle guarding the exit from the bladder becomes weak due to low oestrogen levels. Sometimes urine escapes from the bladder on laughing, coughing or carrying a heavy weight. This is called stress incontinence and it is due to increased pressure inside the abdomen squeezing urine from the bladder. With any or all of these symptoms you may have genital dryness and itching. Vaginal soreness, particularly during or after intercourse because the vagina fails to lubricate, is also common among menopausal and postmenopausal women.

NIGHT SWEATS SELF-HELP

The following simple measures can relieve symptoms.

- *Keep your bedroom temperature fairly cool, and leave a window open if you feel it is safe to do so.*

- *Avoid nightclothes and bed linen made of synthetic fabrics such as nylon and polyester; cotton will be more comfortable.*

- *Keep a bowl of tepid water and a sponge by your bed so that you can cool yourself down easily. Never use cold water; it can cause you to overheat. Allow the water to evaporate on your skin – as it does so it will take the heat from your skin and make you feel cooler.*

VITAMIN E

Although there's no proof of its effectiveness, you could try taking vitamin E, which may help the proper functioning of blood and aid the production of sex hormones.

The recommended dose is one thousand international units (IU) a day and you should not exceed that. Vitamin E appears to work more effectively when it is taken with vitamins B and C (for good food sources, see p. 36). It is also absorbed better in the presence of fats, so vitamin E supplements should be taken at the end of meals. Avoid vitamin E if you suffer from high blood pressure, diabetes or heart problems.

VAGINAL AND URINARY SELF-HELP

The following simple measures can relieve symptoms.

• *For urinary problems of any kind, it is extremely important to keep the bladder flushed out. Try to drink at least two litres (approximately four pints) of fluid a day, especially if you are prone to cystitis (see pp. 85–86).*

• *Keep your urine alkaline since this discourages infections. There are many proprietary products on sale in pharmacies that will alkalinize your urine, or you can drink milk, or take antacids (but not regularly). Try also drinking cranberry juice every morning.*

• *Vaginal dryness, soreness, itchiness or pain during intercourse are greatly relieved with a vaginal moisturizing gel, known as aqueous gel; it's available over the counter and has adhesive properties that helps it to stick to the vaginal walls. Moisturizing the vagina also helps to discourage vaginal infections. A single application of aqueous gel may last up to four days, and it can be used twice a week.*

• *Wearing loose cotton underwear should help prevent irritation of the urogenital tract. You should also avoid using perfumed additives in your bath.*

MEDICAL TREATMENT

Treatment consists almost entirely of HRT, whether in the form of tablets, skin patches or locally applied creams. A vaginal cream is an excellent way of treating vaginal thinness and dryness, stress incontinence and urgent, frequent urination. Recent research has shown that HRT also reduces the frequency of cystitis attacks.

COMPLEMENTARY THERAPY

Herbs that may relieve urinary symptoms include buchu, cornsilk and uva-ursi, which has some antiseptic properties. Goldenseal may also be useful since it is believed to have some anti-infective properties.

EXERCISE AND SEX

Vigorous exercise, such as swimming and cycling, brings blood, oxygen and nutrients to the pelvic area, and keeps tissues healthy. Regular sex or masturbation can do the same thing – loving caresses and erotic massage can also improve circulation to the pelvic area and encourage good vaginal lubrication.

Doing Kegel exercises will strengthen all the pelvic muscles, but particularly those of the urethra, vagina and anus. You can locate the muscles that you use in Kegel exercises by stopping the flow of urine midstream when you're emptying your bladder. Kegel exercises can be done at any time and in any place: all you have to do is draw up the vaginal muscles, hold for a count of five, and then relax. Repeat this process five times. You should do the whole routine at least ten times a day.

MUSCLE AND JOINT SYMPTOMS

General fatigue at the menopause may be profound. Besides underused muscles and joints, there are other causes of chronic fatigue not necessarily connected with the menopause, such as low blood sugar, anaemia and an underactive thyroid gland. Ask your doctor to check all of these if you are experiencing disabling fatigue.

MEDICAL TREATMENT

HRT rapidly relieves the joint stiffness caused by oestrogen deficiency and it maintains muscle strength and the health of ligaments. Although HRT will not reverse the wear and tear in joints, which is called osteoarthritis, it does appear to be beneficial in treating rheumatoid arthritis, in which collagen is lost.

COMPLEMENTARY THERAPY

If you are suffering from stiff and swollen joints, a poultice made with cayenne pepper may be helpful. Other herbal remedies include alfalfa, sarsaparilla, feverfew and white willow. Juniper, rosemary and lavender essential oils may relieve pain when diluted with a base oil and used in a local massage or compress, and the homeopathic remedy Rhus. Tox. may also help.

HAIR, NAILS AND SKIN

With lowered levels of oestrogen, many changes occur. These are due in part to the disintegration of collagen fibres and a weakening of the protein, elastin, which gives connective tissue its strength and suppleness.
- Skin: dryness or oiliness, wrinkles, flaking, bruises easily, wounds heal slowly, patches of brown pigmentation, prominent veins.
- Nails: brittleness, white spots, splinter haemorrhages.
- Gums: bleeding and sponginess, recession leaving tooth roots exposed, infection and periodontal disease, which causes bad breath.
- Hair: dullness, dryness, oiliness, split ends, poor growth, thin patches, dermatitis of the scalp, dandruff.
- Mouth and tongue: cracks on the corners of the lips, mouth ulcers that are slow to heal, the tongue may become thinner and smoother, and the sides scalloped.

MEDICAL TREATMENT

The skin responds quickly to HRT by becoming thicker and better toned. Most women report a change in their skin tone within a few weeks of beginning treatment.

HRT also provides relief from formication (an intense tingling that can feel as if insects are crawling across the skin), and restores hair to its former health. Thinning and baldness will be halted and hair will regain its spring and bounce (although oestrogen cannot stimulate the growth of new hair follicles). Tongue soreness and mouth dryness also benefit from HRT; shrunken gums may fill out, nails become less brittle, the tendency to bruise lessens and cuts and wounds will heal faster.

MUSCLE AND JOINT SELF-HELP

Muscles lose their bulk, strength and coordination, and joints become stiff when collagen begins to disintegrate at the menopause.

- *If you keep your muscles strong with regular exercise you will be more agile and, if you do trip up, muscle strength and coordination will help you to fall with less impact.*

- *If you have rheumatoid arthritis or osteoarthritis, ask your doctor about self-help aids for use in the home.*

FACE AND SKIN SELF-HELP

The following simple measures can help protect your face and skin.

- *Keep your skin moisturized. Avoid soap and use cleansing lotions instead.*

- *Take special care of your nails. Give yourself a manicure and pedicure every eight weeks.*

- *Rinse mouth and tongue ulcers at once with salty water, or use a proprietary ointment.*

- *Guard your skin from the sun. Avoid direct sun at all times, and when you go out in sunny weather, wear a sun block. If possible, limit your exposure to the early and late parts of the day.*

SEXUAL SELF-HELP

The following simple measures can help make sex more enjoyable and fulfilling.

- *Before sex, put some sterile, water-soluble jelly on your vaginal entrance. You may want to put a small amount inside your vagina and on your partner's penis. Water-based jellies are better than oil-based ones because they are less likely to promote infections, and they will not cause the rubber of a condom to perish.*

- *Avoid douches and perfumed talcum powder, toilet paper, bath oils and foams, which can irritate the vagina.*

- *Avoid washing the inside of your labia with soap since it will dry the skin.*

- *Avoid remedies for genital itchiness that contain an antihistamine or perfume.*

- *Spend longer on foreplay to give your body more time to produce its own lubrication. Gentle massage of the breasts, belly, thighs and genitals can be extremely erotic and aid lubrication. Menopausal women can usually lubricate as well as younger women; it simply takes them longer.*

- *Research shows that regular sex or masturbation may help to keep the vagina lubricated. The muscle contractions that occur during orgasm, and the increased blood flow during sex, also seem to exercise the vagina, helping it retain its premenopausal state.*

DIET AND EXERCISE

The health of the skin, nails and hair depends largely on a diet rich in vitamins, minerals and trace elements (see side columns, pp. 36 and 37). It is essential that you have a sufficient intake of the vitamins A, B, C and E, as well as potassium, zinc, magnesium, bioflavonoids, iron, calcium and essential fatty acids. In particular you need foods that are rich in the B vitamins, especially B^1, B^2, B^3, B^6, B^{12} and folic acid.

SEXUAL SYMPTOMS

A common myth about the menopause is that it marks the beginning of a woman's sexual decline. Nothing could be further from the truth. The majority of women can continue to experience sexual pleasure well into old age, indeed as long as their health remains good. Some women even report that their sexual enjoyment starts to increase after the menopause. One of the most common sexual problems after the menopause is lack of lubrication. The vaginal lining may actually crack and bleed and this makes penetration painful, and sometimes impossible. In youth, blood flows quickly to the genitals during arousal, causing swelling and sensitivity to touch. After the menopause there is less engorgement of the clitoris, the vagina and the vulva, leading to subdued arousal.

Sexual desire can also be diminished by certain drugs, such as tranquillizers, muscle relaxants, antidepressants, amphetamines, diuretics, antihypertensives and hormones. Alcohol, smoking, coffee, overwork, tension and depression have the same effect. Women who have had a hysterectomy or surgical removal of the ovaries may also experience a diminished enjoyment of sex and a reduced ability to reach orgasm.

MEDICAL TREATMENT

All forms of HRT should relieve vaginal dryness and soreness if an adequate dose of oestrogen is given. If vaginal symptoms are your only menopausal problem, you could ask your doctor for a vaginal oestrogen cream or pessary. It takes about four weeks of treatment with oestrogen before the physical symptoms affecting the vagina begin to improve. A low-dose testosterone product can be used to increase sex drive.

COMPLEMENTARY THERAPY

Herbs have always been used to treat low sex drive, although some, such as nutmeg, have been found to irritate the urogenital system and should be avoided. Traditional Indian medicine uses the saffron crocus as an aphrodisiac, and the bark of an African tree, *yohimbine*, is the source of several drugs used to treat impotence.

INSOMNIA

If you are feeling depressed or anxious, or are suffering from night sweats, it can become difficult to get to sleep, and common to wake early in the morning. Eventually, a good night's rest can become a rarity.

Women who have normal levels of oestrogen fall asleep faster than women who don't and spend more time in the deepest (dream) stage of sleep; they also feel more refreshed when they wake up. Dreaming seems to be particularly important for the feeling of rest and renewal that comes from sleeping. Without oestrogen, we can sleep for a whole night but still feel tired on waking.

MEDICAL TREATMENT

Before deciding on an appropriate medication, you and your doctor should make a correct diagnosis of your insomnia. If menopausal symptoms, such as night sweats or anxiety, are preventing you from sleeping, then HRT will cure your insomnia. If your sleeplessness is caused by a medical complaint or emotional problem unrelated to the menopause, you may be prescribed sleeping tablets. Although these are sometimes useful to help you through a traumatic life event, such as bereavement or divorce, you may suffer from withdrawal effects, particularly if you take sleeping tablets over a long period of time. Even though nowadays most doctors prescribe short-acting benzodiazepines, which are quickly eliminated by the body, you should be wary of taking sleeping pills unless it is absolutely necessary.

COMPLEMENTARY THERAPY

Valerian root is an age-old herbal remedy to induce sleep and its sedative effect can be very therapeutic during the menopause. Insomnia can also be helped by night-time teas made with herbs such as catnip, camomile and hops.

INSOMNIA SELF-HELP

The following simple measures can relieve symptoms.

● *Rid yourself of night sweats or bring them under control (see pp. 24–25) so that you can sleep undisturbed.*

● *Take a long walk or some other form of aerobic exercise an hour before bedtime; the quality of your sleep should improve noticeably.*

● *Read a good book, or a chapter from a good book; getting "out" of yourself will help you relax, which should make it easier to go to sleep.*

● *Warm milk at bedtime works for many insomniacs. This may be due to the action of calcium on the nerves.*

MONITORING YOUR WEIGHT

Following the simple steps below will tell you whether you need to lose weight.

• *How do you know whether you are too fat or too thin? Consider your body shape. Check to see if you carry more weight around your stomach and waist than around your hips and thighs; the former carries a greater risk of heart disease (see column, right).*

• *Stand relaxed and measure your waist at its narrowest point, then measure your hips at their widest point. Divide your waist measurement by your hip measurement to obtain your waist-to-hip ratio. Ratios above 0.8 are linked to a greater risk of diabetes, heart disease, high blood pressure, osteoporosis and arthritis. If you fall into this category, discuss it with your doctor.*

• *If your waist-to-hip ratio is not in the high risk category, you were not overweight before the menopause and are no more than 6–8 kg (13–18 lb) more after it, then there is no health advantage in reducing your weight. Eating a variety of healthy foods and exercising regularly will allow your body to settle down to its natural weight (see pp. 36–41).*

WEIGHT GAIN

Some postmenopausal women strive to maintain their premenopausal weight. Medically this is quite unsound: the weight that you may gain at the menopause is due to a slower metabolism – something that affects both men and women as they grow older – and a decline in oestrogen levels, which also affects the way that fat is distributed. It's important to be realistic and understand that changes in body shape happen to all postmenopausal women.

Middle-aged women who are 3.5–4.5 kg (8–12 lb) underweight live less long than those who are 3.5–4.5 kg (8–12 lb) overweight. I don't wish to encourage any woman to become obese, but I do wish to free her from the pressure to be thin.

MEDICAL TREATMENT

Unless you are so overweight that your health is being affected, weight gain requires no medical treatment. But if your weight is posing a threat to your health, and you have other risk factors for heart disease, such as high blood pressure and you smoke, it's sensible to ask your doctor to recommend a diet and to supervise your weight loss programme. Some women resort to surgical techniques such as liposuction in an attempt to lose weight, but this should be regarded as an extreme measure. Other women may benefit from counselling.

DIET AND EXERCISE

If your weight is over the recommended weight for your height and age, these tips may help you to lose weight:
• Drink a glass of water before you start to eat. This will make you feel more satiated at the end of a meal.
• Put your food on a small plate. This controls the amount you can reasonably eat at one sitting.
• The more time you take eating food, the more satisfied you'll feel. People who over-eat usually eat quickly, don't taste the food and eat more in order to feel satisfied.
• Exercising an hour or so before a meal is a potent appetite suppressant.
• Eat your largest meal early in the day, when you have more waking time to burn up the calories you've eaten. Avoid eating a large meal late in the evening – sleeping during the night does not burn off many calories.

HEART PROBLEMS

Problems with the heart are rare in premenopausal women because of the presence of oestrogen, but after the menopause, heart disease becomes as common in women as it is in men. The warning symptom of heart disease is angina, which is a symptom of insufficient oxygen reaching the heart muscle. It is experienced as a crushing pain in the middle of the chest brought on by effort or physical exertion and alleviated by rest. Without rest, the pain can worsen and radiate up into the neck and teeth, and down into the arm (usually the left arm but occasionally the right). Eventually the pain will become so bad that you will be forced to stop what you are doing. Angina can start within five years of the menopause; you should take any chest pain seriously and go to your doctor for a cardiac check-up.

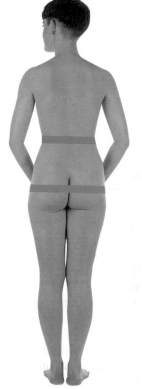

PREMENOPAUSE

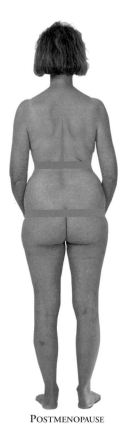

POSTMENOPAUSE

How body shape is related to heart disease
Before the menopause, the waist-to-hip ratio is generally less than 0.8 and there is a correspondingly low risk of heart disease. After the menopause, fat distribution changes and the risk of heart disease increases. You can assess your risk by dividing your waist measurement by your hip measurement. If the resulting figure is over 0.8 you fall into a higher risk group for heart disease.
For example:
74 cm (29 in) ÷ 99 cm (39 in) = 0.74 (low risk)
81 cm (32 in) ÷ 99 cm (39 in) = 0.81 (higher risk)

KEY

■ WAIST MEASUREMENT

■ HIP MEASUREMENT

HEART PROBLEMS SELF-HELP

These simple measures can help the health of your heart.

• *Try to avoid risk factors such as smoking and obesity. If you are carrying more than a few extra kilograms or pounds, it will help to lose weight.*

• *Knowing how to keep yourself calm during times of stress and anxiety is important (see columns, pp. 41 and 42). Try to practise deep breathing and relaxation techniques.*

Other symptoms relating to heart health are palpitations and shortness of breath on exertion. You may find that normal exercise leaves you unusually breathless and climbing several flights of stairs gives you a pumping, fluttery feeling in your chest.

If you are suffering from other symptoms, such as dizziness, headaches or blurred vision, have your blood pressure checked since you may have hypertension.

MEDICAL TREATMENT

There is a wide range of drugs to treat heart conditions, including hypotensives, betablockers, diuretics, cardiac stimulants and coronary vasodilators. Angina can be controlled by taking a coronary vasodilator whenever you have an attack; this dilates the blood vessels so that more blood and oxygen can get to the heart. The tablet is placed underneath the tongue and rapidly dissolves into the bloodstream, giving almost immediate relief. You can even take one of these tablets before exercising to prevent angina in the first place.

If you have high cholesterol, your doctor will probably prescribe drugs to lower it and reduce the possibility of serious heart complications. If you do suffer from heart disease, treatments include an artificial pacemaker, a coronary bypass operation or balloon angioplasty, depending on the type of heart condition you have.

The role of oestrogen in preventing heart disease is controversial. It used to be thought that taking oestrogen helped to prevent the onset of heart disease in women, but a recent study in the US appears to contradict this. For the moment at least, women with a history of heart disease who wish to begin or continue HRT should thoroughly discuss their personal risks and benefits from the therapy with their doctors before making any decison.

DIET AND EXERCISE

Try to limit the amount of salt you eat from all sources, including processed food. You can reduce your blood pressure by several points if you eliminate salt.

• Recent research seems to confirm that garlic improves cardiovascular health, although many doctors remain sceptical. You can eat garlic in meals or take garlic pearls, which are odourless.

• Regular exercise is the only way to strengthen a weak heart, and it will help to reduce high blood pressure. However, if you have heart problems, you should consult your doctor before you start exercising to ensure that you do not go beyond your physical capabilities.

EMOTIONAL SYMPTOMS

Tension, anxiety, depression, listlessness, irritability, tearfulness and mood swings can occur at any age, but they rarely occur together, or as frequently, as they do during the menopause. This is because the centres in the brain that control your sense of well-being, a positive state of mind and a feeling of control and tranquillity are affected by the absence of oestrogen, so for many women menopausal mood changes resemble a roller-coaster ride. Some women describe subtle sensations such as trembling, fluttering, unease and discomfort. Other women find that severe feelings of anxiety or panic can arise with little provocation; tasks that they used to be able to tackle easily can leave them in total disarray. Mood swings from elation to despondency are common, and patience is quickly exhausted. If you have these symptoms, the future may look bleak, your loss of self-esteem is precipitous, and you may feel truly depressed. But taking oestrogen supplements in the form of HRT can cause a dramatic return to normality.

For some women, the emotional troubles they experience around the menopause may be due mainly to night sweats interrupting their sleep. Tired people are often irritable, anxious and short-tempered. If you have this problem, try the self-help tips on page 25.

MEDICAL TREATMENT

The mainstay of treatment for emotional symptoms is HRT. Studies from all over the world show that after a short period (between two weeks and two months), HRT can bring about a significant decline in anxiety and depression. Oestrogen even lifts the mood in non-depressed, healthy young women. It acts through several well-known antidepressive mechanisms in the brain, on which other antidepressant drugs act. The calming effect of oestrogen is at least the equivalent of tranquillizers such as diazepam and chlorodiazepoxide, and oestrogen can be a great deal healthier to take.

EMOTIONAL SELF-HELP

You'll be better able to cope with emotional symptoms if you follow these guidelines.

• *Share your feelings with your partner. Severe mood swings and irritability can distance you from your partner and, occasionally, can jeopardize a relationship. Several studies show that partners are keen to understand menopausal symptoms and would prefer to have insight into potential problems before the onset of the menopause.*

• *Think about joining a self-help group, or even starting one yourself. Women who go to these groups may be better able to deal with depression.*

• *Twenty to thirty minutes of strenuous exercise results in the release of endorphins, which are the body's own "feel-good" chemicals. This can lift the mood and produce an "exercise high" that lasts up to eight hours. Exercise can also benefit hot flushes and night sweats, which is helpful if this is the root cause of your depression.*

• *Yoga, relaxation techniques and meditation all promote tranquillity and combat anxiety and tension.*

INTELLECTUAL SELF-HELP

Any sort of work or studying will go a long way to preserve your intellectual ability.

It's never too late to get a job, although many women in their menopausal years worry about how to go about finding one. Many evening classes, colleges and universities offer courses in a range of subjects, including employment retraining.

MEDICAL TREATMENT

Most intellectual skills improve as soon as you start to take HRT. You feel more self-confident about making decisions, more assertive, better able to concentrate, and you are less forgetful.

Very sophisticated research shows that normal oestrogen levels are responsible for memory. Oestrogen exerts an extremely subtle effect on the memory process. It improves our verbal memory and the way we store information; it affects the way we relate our past experiences to present situations by helping us to have realistic expectations; it helps our working memory; and it helps us to process information efficiently, in fact, to put two and two together and make four. Current research into HRT and Alzheimer's disease looks very promising. Women with a family history of Alzheimer's would be advised to take HRT if suitable.

COMPLEMENTARY THERAPY

Herbs that may have a calming effect are passion flower and valerian root, taken as a tea or a tincture. Passion flower helps insomnia and elevates the levels of serotonin in the blood, which creates a feeling of well-being. Taking a bath with an infusion of your favourite herbs can also be therapeutic.

Menopausal depression and stress may be alleviated by ginger root, cayenne pepper, dandelion root and Siberian ginseng. They may work because they contain essential nutrients, for instance, dandelion root contains magnesium, potassium and vitamin E; cayenne pepper contains a high level of magnesium and bioflavonoids. Ginseng can have a tonic effect, and Siberian ginseng and liquorice root are also considered to be very effective in combatting lassitude and depression.

INTELLECTUAL SYMPTOMS

Forgetfulness is one of the most common symptoms that menopausal women complain of, and they may experience it long before they stop menstruating. You may forget where you put something, you may miss appointments and things that used to be easy to remember can suddenly require enormous effort. The ability to concentrate can also become difficult. These problems combined can make it hard to carry out work that involves complex assessments and major decision-making. Even minor decisions can sometimes be quite paralysing.

DIET AND EXERCISE

Relatively little research has been done on the effects that nutrients have on intellectual processes, but there is some evidence that vitamins B^1 and B^{12} and minerals such as calcium and potassium may contribute to brain health. These are easy to incorporate into a normal healthy diet (for food sources of vitamins and minerals, see columns, pp. 36 and 37), but bear in mind that most vitamins need to be taken in conjunction with other vitamins and minerals in order to be absorbed by the body.

Regular exercise also helps you feel more alert and less sluggish, and can improve concentration too. A brisk walk in the fresh air every day for at least 20 minutes will tone you up mentally as well as physically.

CHAPTER 3

A HEALTHY MENOPAUSE

Monitoring and maintaining your health is the key to continuing a healthy, happy and active life. Observing and reading the messages your body sends, and responding sensitively to them, bring a real sense of achievement as well as well-being. And there is simply no doubt about it: it is not difficult to enjoy natural good health. Eating healthy food *does* make you feel better; controlling your weight *does* make you look better; and keeping fit *does* make you more energetic and alert. What's more, any efforts you make quickly become apparent, giving you the incentive to continue the good work.

*You can get all the vitamins
you need from fresh foods.*

Vitamin A *Carrots, spinach,
turnips, apricots, liver, sweet
potatoes, cantaloupe melon.*

Folic Acid *Green leafy
vegetables, nuts, peas, beans,
liver and kidney. Folic acid
prevents spina bifida and
hydrocephalus in the unborn
child. Remember that although
the menopause signals the end
of fertility, you can still become
pregnant for up to two years
after your last menstrual period.*

Vitamin B 3 *Meat and
poultry, fish, pulses, whole
wheat, bran.*

Vitamin B 6 *Meat and
poultry, fish, bananas,
wholegrain cereals, dairy
products. Vitamin B 6 is useful
in treating symptoms of PMS.*

Vitamin B 12 *Fish, poultry,
eggs and milk, B 12-enriched
soya produce (no vegetable
contains B 12). Vitamin B 12
prevents pernicious anaemia.*

Vitamin C *Citrus fruits,
strawberries, broccoli, green
peppers.*

Vitamin D *Oily fish, fortified
cereals and bread, fortified
margarine, (sunlight).*

Vitamin E *Vegetable oils,
green leafy vegetables, cereals,
dried beans, wholegrains,
wholemeal bread.*

GOOD NUTRITION

As you get older, your digestive tract becomes less efficient and digestion can take longer; your body no longer finds it as easy to cope with foods that contain a lot of calories but little nourishment. Although you need fewer calories than you did when you were younger, you still require the same amount of vitamins and minerals. The healthiest diet during the menopause, therefore, is one that consists of unprocessed fresh foods, such as wholegrains, vegetables, fruits, fish, seafood, some oils and eggs. A whole range of healthy foods is now widely available in every high street, so it has never been easier to experiment. Concentrate on building up a regular diet of unprocessed, high-grade carbohydrates to which protein can be added as a "condiment".

As your body's metabolism and chemical reactions slow down, an adequate intake of vitamins and minerals is essential; eating the right diet can have a powerful and beneficial effect on menopausal symptoms, making you independent of doctors and drugs.

Start to cut down on the amount of meat in your diet, and try to eat more rice, beans, vegetables and pasta. Root vegetables may help the body to produce progesterone and soya foods may increase bone mineral content in post-menopausal women. Avoid too much coffee and alcohol. Vitamin D is recommended where a deficiency may exist (vitamin D is always taken with calcium).

A certain amount of fat, however, is needed for functions that cannot be performed by any other nutrient, and essential fatty acids are necessary for the metabolism of calcium, for instance, and cannot be manufactured by the body. The best forms of fat are those found in whole natural foods, such as vegetable oils and fish oils. Fats to avoid are saturated fats, that is, fats that are solid at room temperature; these include butter and lard, and certain vegetable oils, such as coconut or palm oil found in processed foods.

Fermented milk products, for example yogurt, can be particularly effective at encouraging calcium absorption. Even those who have problems digesting whole-milk products can usually tolerate fermented ones because they are partially predigested.

REDUCING SUGAR

Most people eat too much sugar. These guidelines will help you to cut down.

• Reduce your intake of convenience foods, relishes, ketchup, cakes, biscuits, sweets and fizzy drinks, all of which have high levels of sugar.

• Avoid refined carbohydrate foods, such as white flour, white bread, white sugar or white rice, which are low in fibre and can contribute to obesity.

• When cooking, try to cut the amount of sugar in a recipe by about one-third; this won't spoil the taste at all.

• Satisfy cravings for chocolate and other sweet foods with healthier alternatives, like fresh fruit and fruit juice.

• Eat more fibre. A high-fibre diet will fill you up so that you are less likely to want a snack (see below).

• If you have a sweet tooth, substitute a healthier sweetener, such as honey, which also has a sweeter taste than sugar, weight for weight. You can also substitute fruit for sugar in pastries, cakes and biscuits.

REDUCING SALT

Follow these guidelines to reduce your salt consumption.

• Cut down on prepared foods, such as hamburgers, salad dressings, hot dogs, pizzas and French fries. If you're buying these foods, always look for brands that have no added salt.

• Avoid adding salt to already cooked food. Fruits, vegetables, meat and grains contain all the salt you will ever need in your diet.

• Enhance natural salt in foods by using flavourings such as garlic, herbs, spices and lemon.

• Substitute potassium-based salt for table salt – it's healthy and doesn't exacerbate high blood pressure or heart disease.

• Try seasoning vegetables with powdered seaweeds, such as kelp or nori (available from healthfood shops). They're rich in essential iodine and many trace elements.

INCREASING FIBRE

The following simple measures (see p. 38) will help you to increase your fibre intake. Make the transition to raw, high-fibre food slowly, and don't worry if it takes a few months to change your dietary and eating habits.

ESSENTIAL MINERALS

You can get all the minerals you need from fresh foods.

Calcium *Milk and milk products, dark-green leafy vegetables, citrus fruits, dried peas and beans.*

Magnesium *Green leafy vegetables, nuts, soya beans, wholegrain cereals.*

Potassium *Orange juice, bananas, dried fruits, peanut butter, meat.*

Zinc *Meat, liver, eggs, poultry, seafood.*

Iron *Nuts, liver, red meats, egg yolk, green leafy vegetables, dried fruits.*

Iodine *Seafood, fish, seaweed such as nori and kelp.*

Chromium *Meat, cheese, wholegrains, breads.*

Selenium *Seafood, meat, wholegrain cereals.*

Manganese *Nuts, fruits and vegetables, wholegrain cereals.*

Bioflavonoids *All citrus fruits, especially the pulp and pith, soya products.*

POSITIVE EATING

Although you need fewer calories at this time of your life, your body's nutritional needs remain the same.

• *Calorie counting may be too time-consuming for anyone to maintain in the long term, so it's much better to concentrate on eating a diet that is well balanced and contains no "empty" high-calorie foods such as sugar and fat.*

• *You can change not only what you eat, but how you eat. Eating five or even six small meals at regular intervals is very effective in weight control because each time you eat, you use energy in digestion. Small, frequent meals also stop blood sugar levels dropping, which can be accompanied by cravings for food.*

• Switch to high-fibre bread.
• Have high-fibre cereal for your breakfast.
• Eat high-fibre soups such as bean, lentil or sweetcorn.
• Include different types of beans and peas when you are making green salads.
• Use dark-green salad leaves such as spinach, rocket and curly endive instead of pale iceberg lettuce.
• Eat bean dips with raw vegetables or wholewheat pitta bread.
• Use unprocessed flour, nuts and sesame seeds in your standard recipes, where appropriate.
• Snack on wholegrain crackers and dried fruits.
• Eat wholemeal muffins instead of cakes and biscuits.

HIGH STRESS FOODS

Sugar, caffeine, alcohol and other substances contribute to various menopausal problems. High-stress foods contain few nutrients and, in some cases, they may be addictive; try substituting the healthier alternatives given in the chart below. In addition, avoid black pepper, prepared dishes containing monosodium glutamate (MSG) and very hot spices such as chilli (which worsen hot flushes), or cut the amount by half.

HEALTHY ALTERNATIVES FOR HIGH-STRESS FOODS

HIGH-STRESS FOODS	HEALTHY ALTERNATIVES
135 g (4 oz) white flour	135 g (4 oz) wholewheat flour
1 square chocolate	1 square of carob or 1 tablespoon powdered carob
1 tablespoon coffee	1 tablespoon decaffeinated coffee
½ teaspoon salt	½ teaspoon of one of the following: potassium salt substitute, yeast extract, dried basil, tarragon or oregano
125 ml (4 fl oz) wine	125 ml (4 fl oz) low-alcohol wine
250 ml (8 fl oz) beer	250 ml (8 fl oz) low-alcohol beer
250 ml (8 fl oz) milk	250 ml (8 fl oz) soya milk
150 g (5 oz) sugar	One of the following: ¼ cup molasses, ½ cup honey, ½ cup maple syrup, ½ cup barley malt, 2 cups apple juice

WEIGHT CONTROL

Many studies have been carried out to show the differences between people who eat small, frequent meals and those who eat fewer, larger ones. The latter invariably have more body fat than the former. Some dieters find that a diet based on a nibbling pattern helps to prevent hunger pangs, and there is some evidence that this may speed up weight loss.

Try not to go on crash diets or long-term diets that are little more than starvation. The initial weight loss may be impressive but less than half of this will be fat; most will be water, and it could include some of your precious body protein. A diet that restricts total calorie intake to under a thousand calories is only just adequate. Very strict diets, those around 500 calories, cannot provide all the required nutrients for an adult woman.

A crash diet offers severely obese people a chance to lose up to one to two kilograms (three to six pounds) per week. However, there is much research to show that towards the end of a long period of this kind of dieting, the rate of weight loss decelerates and the weight starts to go back on when normal eating patterns are resumed. In other words, the body adapts to starvation.

The fewer calories we give the body, the less it needs, until it can finally get by on fewer than 300 calories a day. A return to normal eating patterns will cause an inevitable increase in weight as body stores of glycogen are replaced; this is extremely depressing if you have made a great effort to shed excess weight. It is common for a person coming off a starvation diet to go on eating binges and find herself on a treadmill of intermittent starving and bingeing that is extremely damaging to her health and self-image.

CHANGING MEAL PATTERNS

Rather than having a set menu for breakfast, lunch and dinner, think in terms of what type of food you would like to eat and how much time and energy you have to prepare it. For example, choose to cook a more elaborate meat meal at the weekend when you have plenty of time both to prepare and eat, and a nutritious but simple-to-make soup or pasta meal during weekday evenings, when you have less energy to devote to either.

WATCHING YOUR WEIGHT

Your digestive system will probably prefer a nibbling pattern diet, particularly if you suffer from indigestion or a peptic ulcer. Try the following tips to help curb your appetite.

• *Drink 250 ml (half a pint) of water before you start to eat. This will make you feel more satisfied at the end of a meal.*

• *Serve your meal on a small plate. This controls the amount you can eat at any one meal.*

• *Eat slowly; you will be more satisfied and you will be less likely to over-eat.*

• *Taking exercise an hour or so before a meal can help suppress your appetite.*

• *Avoid eating large meals late in the evening; sleeping during the night does not burn off very many calories.*

HOW REGULAR EXERCISE HELPS

Taking regular exercise has many physical and mental benefits. It gives you:

• *A reduced risk of heart disease.*

• *A lower chance of developing diabetes mellitus.*

• *Maintenance of muscle tone and strength.*

• *Higher levels of the healthy type of cholesterol in the blood.*

• *Healthier bones and less chance of developing osteoporosis later in life.*

• *A more efficient immune system to fight disease.*

• *Reduced body fat.*

• *Better appetite control.*

• *Increased mental agility.*

• *Fewer headaches.*

• *Improved sleep quality.*

• *Flexible joints.*

KEEPING FIT

Without doubt, exercise is the menopausal woman's best friend in that it allows you to control your body and emotions by using your internal resources. Each time that you take exercise, your adrenal glands are stimulated to convert the male hormone androstenedione into oestrogen. A minimum of four 30-minute exercise sessions each week will help to keep your body producing a little oestrogen. As you become older, your cardio-respiratory fitness, your strength and your flexibility all begin to decline. For people who remain active, however, these things decrease at a lower rate (an average of five percent per decade after the age of about 20, as opposed to nine percent per decade).

Long-term exercise also means that you will have stronger bones and a lower risk of osteoporosis than non-exercisers. Although every woman is different, most of us lose 25–35 percent of our bone mass by the time we reach the age of 65. Bone loss begins around the age of 35, proceeds slowly up to the menopause, and then accelerates during the five to seven years after the menopause, when oestrogen levels are low.

Regular exercise may also have a significant effect on our mental agility by increasing the amount of oxygen supplied to the brain. In a comparison between sedentary older women and older women who exercised regularly, after four months the latter group processed information faster in tests. Exercise can also prevent our reaction times from slowing down.

WHICH TYPE OF EXERCISE?

The type of exercise that you take obviously depends largely on resources, how much time you have to devote to exercise and your own personal preference. Nowadays there is a wide range of opportunities available, and not only in sports centres and fitness classes. If you need or prefer to exercise in your own home, there are many excellent exercise videos and other publications on the market that will show you the best ways to preserve your muscle strength and tone.

You may prefer a sport such as tennis, badminton or squash, all of which offer the added attraction of meeting and socializing with people. Likewise, joining an aerobics or exercise class can provide a social aspect that may encourage you to exercise regularly. Less rigorous and more traditional forms of exercise, such as walking and swimming, offer viable alternatives, and will keep the body fit and supple. Unfortunately, you cannot "store" the benefits of exercise; it must be ongoing to confer its many benefits (see column, left).

THINKING POSITIVELY

The first step towards taking charge of your life and managing your menopause is to take charge of your body. You need to play an active role with all of your medical and health providers. Be aware of all your options and exercise them in order to eliminate as many health problems as you can. The strategy you choose to deal with any menopausal symptoms you may suffer from is up to you. You could decide to try self-help measures, for instance, or complementary medicine such as herbal remedies or homeopathy. Alternatively, you may feel that your symptoms warrant conventional medical help.

To achieve these goals, you need to have a firm sense of your own self-worth and optimism about the future, and you must be prepared to make an effort. As soon as you start to take control of your menopausal symptoms, your health and sense of well-being will benefit greatly.

The second step towards taking charge of your life and managing your menopause is to take charge of your mind. As with your body, you need to be positive in your attitude and prepared to make a real effort to get what you want from both your family and friends, and from medical and other professionals with whom you come into contact. Try to keep in mind positive statements such as "Femininity does not have to equal fertility", and remember that the menopause is not the beginning of the end; it's the beginning of the rest of your life.

While health and vigour during the menopausal years depend a great deal on following a good diet and taking plenty of regular exercise, these are by no means the only resources you have to draw upon. Rest, relaxation and a variety of leisure activities will help you keep active and mentally alert. You also need self-affirming thoughts to maintain your self-confidence and prevent self-criticism. Never allow yourself to think that you are unattractive, lacklustre or out-of-touch.

DEEP MUSCLE RELAXATION

Follow the steps below to relax your body.

1 Find a peaceful place. Lie on your back, or sit in a comfortable chair, and close your eyes.

2 Tense your right hand (or left, if you are left-handed), then let it go loose. Imagine it feels heavy and warm. Repeat with your right forearm, upper arm and shoulder, then move on to the right foot, lower leg, upper leg. Now do exactly the same thing with the left side of your body. By the time you have finished, your hands, arms and legs should feel heavy, relaxed and warm. Allow a few seconds for these feelings to develop and to get used to the sensation.

3 Now relax the muscles around your hips and waist. Let the relaxation flow up the abdomen into the chest. You will find that your breathing starts to slow down.

4 Let the relaxation go into your shoulders, facial and jaw muscles. Pay special attention to the muscles around your eyes and forehead – tense them, then let the frown melt away. Finish by imagining that your forehead feels cool and smooth.

DEEP MENTAL RELAXATION

Follow the steps below to relax your mind.

1 Allow thoughts to associate freely in your head.

2 Stop any recurring negative thoughts by saying "no" to them under your breath, and repeating a firm "no" until they go away.

3 With your eyes closed, imagine a tranquil scene such as a calm blue sea. Whatever you imagine, try to see the colour blue, because this is very therapeutic.

4 Concentrate on your breathing – and make sure it is deep, slow and natural. Follow each breath as you inhale and exhale.

5 By now, you should feel calm and rested. You may find it helpful to repeat a soothing mantra, such as "love", "peace" or "calm".

6 Remind yourself to keep the muscles of your face, eyes and forehead relaxed, and imagine that your forehead is cool and smooth.

STAYING MENTALLY FIT

Without stimulation, our brains will slow down and become feeble (remember that the best mental exercise is work). We can learn a lot by observing the qualities of people whose mental and emotional resilience we admire. The following qualities come from emotional openness, flexibility and self-reliance.

• Independence and recognition of others' independence, privacy and peace.

• Lack of self-pity, so that when a problem arises it is looked at objectively.

• The attitude that nothing is hopeless and problems are there to be solved.

• A sense of inner security rather than security gained from controlling others.

• Taking responsibility for our own mistakes.

• A few close and loving relationships rather than many superficial ones.

• A sense of realism about the goals we set ourselves.

• Being in touch with our emotions and feeling free to express them.

MEMORY MAINTENANCE

You can improve your memory by following the simple measures outlined below.

• When you read a book or magazine article, summarize the plot or the points made in it to a friend.

• When you're going shopping, try to collect as many items as possible without referring to your shopping list.

• If you want to remember several things, do it with a mnemonic – a series of letters forming a word that will act as a memory aid. For example, you can abbreviate tasks such as ironing, making a phone call and typing a letter into the single word, PIT (Phone/Iron/Type).

• If you walk into a room and forget why you're there, go back to where you came from and don't leave until you have remembered.

• If you have lost something, track it down. Write down the last six things you did prior to losing it and where you were for each activity. Draw a grid with what you were doing along one side and where you were along the bottom. The item you've lost lies in one of those squares; check out each one until you come across it.

CHAPTER 4

WHAT IS HRT?

HRT (hormone replacement therapy) aims to correct the deficit of the female hormones, oestrogen and progesterone, that occurs at the menopause. Doctors prescribe these two hormones in a variety of combinations, tailored to suit the individual, to alleviate symptoms such as hot flushes, and to prevent serious health problems, like osteoporosis, that may occur when oestrogen levels decline. This chapter explores the medical issues connected with HRT and describes the methods and types of medication available, including tablets, patches, gels, pessaries and creams. It explains the benefits and disadvantages of each method and helps you to make an informed choice about what is right for you.

WHO CAN USE HRT?

The mainstay of orthodox medical treatment of the menopause is hormone replacement therapy (HRT). This treats the menopause as a hormone deficiency state that can be alleviated by replacing the oestrogen and progesterone that a woman's ageing ovaries no longer secrete in sufficient quantities.

Because of the diverse range of HRT products, and the number of ways in which they can be administered, most women can find an HRT regime that matches their needs and produces few side-effects. However, for women who don't wish to take HRT or have a contraindication to its use (see column, p. 58), alternative medications are available.

IT'S YOUR DECISION

Understanding the benefits of HRT means that you have the knowledge to make an intelligent and informed choice. Only you have the final responsibility for your own health care.

It is important to gather as much information as you can and maintain the motivation to keep yourself in the best possible health. On average, women taking HRT live three to four years longer than their contemporaries. So on balance, not taking HRT seems riskier than taking it.

EXPLAINING HORMONAL MEDICATION

The basis of all HRT regimes is oestrogen; progestogens are added solely to induce a uterine bleed with shedding of the endometrium, or uterine lining. The main way of treating menopausal symptoms is to prescribe oestrogen and progestogen. Several regimes, combinations and forms are available – about 70 in all – so one should suit you. There is also a no-bleed product for women who do not want monthly periods – tibolone (see p.49).

HORMONAL MEDICATION

HRT is a substitute for the female sex hormones oestrogen and progesterone; it is prescribed when the body's levels of female hormones are low, most usually at or after the menopause. Oestrogen is given to maintain the health of the whole female body. Progestogen is generally given because it causes the uterine lining to shed (see column, p. 47), which prevents over-thickening of the lining and cancer of the uterus.

The main oestrogens used in HRT are natural, from plant sources, and are similar to oestradiol, which is produced by the ovaries. Some HRT products contain conjugated equine oestrogen harvested from the urine of pregnant mares. Progestogen is the synthetic form of progesterone. Because natural progesterone is rapidly metabolized by the body, it does not produce a sustained effect when taken in tablet form. However, progesterone as suppositories and intra-vaginal cream (prescription only) is powerful enough to protect the endometrium.

The normal menstrual cycle depends on the sequential production of oestrogen and progesterone (see columns, pp. 14 and 15), so it makes sense to include them in menopausal HRT. Another vital hormone is testosterone, also manufactured by the ovaries; if your ovaries are removed, there will be 50 percent less testosterone in your bloodstream. High levels of oestrogen in HRT can neutralize available testosterone. Much of the female sex drive is attributed to this male hormone, and if you are taking HRT and suffering from a lack of libido, discuss with your doctor the possibility of taking low-dose testosterone as an implant or patch or as tablets.

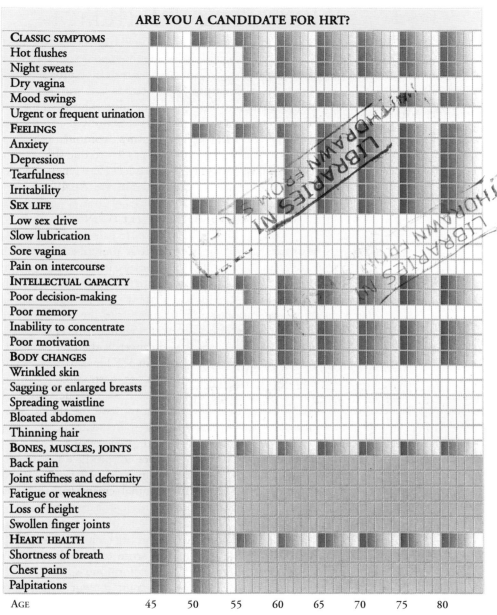

Assessing your candidacy

The orange and yellow panels in this table indicate the maximum number of symptoms you may experience during the menopause and beyond. Find your age along the bottom of the table and look in the list above it to see which symptoms may occur in women of that age.

If you are experiencing two or more of the symptoms marked for your age, then you are highly eligible for HRT. If you have any of the symptoms shown in the orange area, you should discuss your personal risks and benefits from HRT with your doctor.

ABOUT OESTROGEN

Both natural and synthetic forms of oestrogen are available, as are other chemicals that have an oestrogenic effect, but are not, strictly speaking, oestrogens.

Natural oestrogens, derived from human or animal metabolism, are absorbed and excreted by the body more easily than synthetic ones.

Synthetic oestrogens are much more potent than naturally occurring ones and may have some unwanted effects on the body, for example increasing the risk of thrombosis. However, most oestrogens used in HRT are natural and have minimal effects on the body's metabolism. Also, with the wide range of products and potencies available, there is great scope for adjusting the treatment and for finding a product that is suitable for each individual woman.

BENEFITS OF HRT

In this age of preventive medicine, HRT should be hailed as one of the most effective treatments for counteracting long-term disease. Our whole orientation in medicine should be towards prevention rather than cure, and any regime that can cut down on expensive treatments, hospital admissions, and serious disease should be embraced enthusiastically by the medical profession.

Prevention of bowel cancer A recent US study showed that HRT using a combination of oestrogen and progestogen cut the incidence of bowel cancer in menopausal women by 37 percent.

Maintenance of healthy organs, bones and muscles HRT has also proved successful in maintaining the health of all the female reproductive organs. In addition to keeping the tissues of the vagina supple and moist, it can prevent atrophy and thinning of the urinary tract and associated infections and incontinence. Oestrogen contributes to the health, strength and functioning of the bones, muscles and joints and can help to prevent backache – a problem that is common in menopausal women due to osteoporosis of the spine. The general toning effect of HRT on the musculo-skeletal system means a return of strength, stamina and energy.

Improvement in shape There are three ways in which menopausal women can change shape. First, by loss of muscle and ligament strength, second, by the tendency towards male fat distribution on the waist and abdomen, and third, by the loss of height due to osteoporosis. HRT can prevent these changes, which may be partly why some people perceive hormonal medication as youth-promoting. Don't make the mistake of thinking that oestrogen is a dietary or weight-control product – it is not a substitute for good nutrition and exercise.

Increased well-being Beta-endorphins are chemicals from the central nervous system that are associated with a general sense of well-being and euphoria. Reduced beta-endorphins are associated with depression, and it is thought that HRT will increase beta-endorphin levels.

Taking hormones during and after the menopause can directly raise your mood and feelings of self-worth, and alleviate anxiety. Your sense of emotional well-being is likely to improve – the so-called "mental tonic" effect of HRT. You may be able to work better and feel revitalized. Although HRT may alleviate depressed moods, it should not be considered an antidepressant drug.

Relief of menopausal symptoms Women who have hot flushes and night sweats find relief when they take oestrogen, regardless of how they take it (see p. 50). For 98 percent of women, HRT alleviates their symptoms and in over 90 percent, symptoms disappear completely. Very heavy periods can be experienced by women in their late 40s and early 50s. This can be helped by HRT, although severely abnormal bleeding may need assessment by your doctor. Vaginal dryness, soreness and painful intercourse may also be soothed by taking oestrogen. Headaches can become more frequent at the menopause and oestrogen can bring relief.

Your skin will respond to oestrogen by showing increased tone and suppleness. Your hair will be stronger and less prone to dryness and brittleness. Similarly, nails that were brittle and prone to splitting become stronger. Gum recession around the time of menopause can also be alleviated by HRT.

Intellectual problems, for example, an inability to concentrate and difficulty making decisions, tend to disappear within a month or so of taking HRT. In one study, women found relief from panic attacks when they took HRT and received psychotherapy.

The response of the libido to HRT is different for every woman. You may notice an increase in sexual enjoyment, but not necessarily an increase in sex drive. There are low-dose testosterone products that, if taken daily, can bring about a subtle return to sexual vitality without side-effects such as facial hair or lowering of the voice.

Studies from sleep laboratories show that oestrogen changes the proportion of sleep time spent in the rapid eye movement (REM) stage that is characteristic of dreaming. Women may dream more when they take oestrogen and dream less when they are oestrogen deficient. As REM sleep increases, your general state of peacefulness improves and you feel more rested after sleep.

ABOUT PROGESTERONE

The synthetic forms of this naturally occurring hormone are progestin and progestogen.

Originally, HRT consisted only of oestrogen. Progestogen was added when it was found to lower the rate of endometrial (uterine) cancer, and HRT then became the norm for women with a uterus.

Taking progestogen has the disadvantage of a monthly withdrawal bleed. Moreover, a small number of women (about 10–15 percent) experience side-effects, similar to premenstrual syndrome. Progestogen side effects include bloating, fluid retention and depression. See your doctor if these symptoms persist. Fortunately, side-effects subside in about four months for half of all women who take HRT. Your progestogen intake can be reduced by taking it as part of your regime only once every three months (see Cyclical therapy, p. 57).

IF SIDE-EFFECTS PUT YOU OFF...

Only a sixth of the women who start taking HRT continue to take it for one year. Women who drop out are usually anxious about side-effects like weight gain, have read panic stories in the press, or have misconceptions about their treatments.

It is worth remembering that certain side-effects, such as headaches, indigestion and tender breasts, can occur whether you're taking hormones or not.

In several well-controlled studies, women who were told they were taking HRT, but were actually taking a placebo, had as many symptoms as women taking HRT. The important factor seems to be how well informed you are about the side-effects; women who are warned of potential minor problems seem to cope with them better than women who are not so well informed.

YOU AND YOUR DOCTOR

The best doctor–patient relationships are those in which you receive full attention and satisfactory answers. You should be able to visit your doctor with a complete list of questions to which you require answers.

Unfortunately, although this kind of easy relationship should be the norm, some women encounter entrenched conservative opinion that dismisses the menopause as a woman's legacy, requiring neither help nor treatment. If your doctor espouses these attitudes, my advice is to change to a more sympathetic doctor as soon as possible. Don't continue with a doctor with whom you have little rapport. Some of the symptoms you may experience will require you to be open and confident enough to discuss them in intimate detail. If you feel at all inhibited, that doctor is not for you. Remember, doctors are there to help you and provide a service. Shop around until you can find a doctor who really suits you. He or she must be able to tailor your treatment to your individual needs in the light of your medical and gynaecological history. Your doctor should be aware of the possible side-effects of taking hormone replacement therapy, be responsive to your comments about a particular HRT regime, and be able to implement changes in regime or dose until you are happy with your treatment. A doctor who is not well versed in menopausal medicine may not be able to provide quite such an individual service, in which case you should seek specialist advice from menopause or well-woman clinics, or from a gynaecologist.

MANAGING YOUR TREATMENT

Not all women who should get HRT do get it, and many women who are prescribed HRT do not take it for a sufficiently long period to prevent their bone mass declining and to protect them against heart disease. In my opinion, more women should consider trying HRT and more doctors should be prepared to prescribe medication for a four-month trial period. Within four months your doctor can adapt the treatment so that you are able to find the regime that suits your body most. It is worth embarking on the search for the right dose and type of HRT (see pp. 55–56) because it can greatly affect your physical and emotional well-being.

A MONTHLY BLEED?

The first decision for you and your doctor to make when you are contemplating taking HRT is whether or not to have a withdrawal bleed. The consensus of medical opinion is that if you have an intact uterus, you should have a menstrual bleed at regular intervals. Two new approaches – combined continuous therapy (see p. 57) and a progestogenic drug called tibolone – have allowed some women to avoid bleeding altogether, and various menopause experts have been researching three-monthly, rather than monthly withdrawal bleeding (see right).

At one time (and I was involved in this research more than 25 years ago), it was thought that the HRT cycle should be similar to the natural menstrual cycle in that a bleed should take place every month. This was achieved by giving women progestogen for 11–13 days in the second half of the cycle. However, experts currently believe that this is unnecessary and that it is preferable for you to bleed as infrequently as once every three months.

There is also another way of taking HRT, which allows you to take progestogen "on demand". A study in the Netherlands found that the sensitivity of the menopausal endometrium to oestrogens and progestogens is unique to each woman. Research shows that it is possible to monitor growth – induced by oestrogen – of the endometrium, or lining of the uterus, with a technique called vaginosonography, in which an ultrasound picture is used to show the thickness of the uterine lining. This technique can also monitor endometrial shedding after the addition of progestogen to the HRT regime. Vaginosonography enables doctors to find out which type and dose of oestrogen causes the lowest endometrial growth for you, and which type and dose of progestogen causes the best endometrial shedding, with minimal withdrawal bleeding.

Another remarkable and important discovery was that the endometrium could shed itself without withdrawal bleeding after the addition of progestogen; also certain progestogens cause shedding of the endometrium without withdrawal bleeding more often than others. Vaginosonography is available at most specialist centres.

RESEARCH

Doctors involved in research at the Medical Care Programme in Oakland, California, hypothesized that the addition of progestogen every three months instead of every month would be safe.

To evaluate the acceptability of this regime 200 women, who had previously been taking progestogen on a monthly basis, were asked to complete a daily diary and, at the end of the study, to complete a preference questionnaire about which HRT regime they felt suited them best. On the three-monthly regime, the average duration of menstruation was two days longer than it had been formerly. The safety of the treatment was checked by performing a physical examination and carrying out biopsies on the uterine lining at the beginning of treatment and after one year.

The results of the preference questionnaire showed that women preferred the three-monthly progestogen regime to the monthly one, despite the fact that their periods were longer and heavier than before. In addition, a reduction in blood pressure occurred over the year of the study and biopsies of the uterine lining did not reveal any abnormalities, suggesting that a three-monthly progestogen regime is as safe as a monthly one.

This method of taking HRT is available in most parts of the world, so you could discuss it with your doctor.

CHANGING THE DOSE OF HORMONES

Side-effects can occur if you are taking more hormones than your body needs. As a woman's body gets older, it becomes more and more sensitive to female hormones, and a much lower dose is needed for HRT than is needed for contraception.

The aim of HRT is to be effective at the lowest possible dose. For instance, if you are taking conjugated equine oestrogen, it is possible to halve the dose from 1.25 micrograms of oestrogen per day to 0.625 micrograms. Similarly, progestogen could be reduced from 500 micrograms of norethisterone acetate per day to 300 micrograms. Make sure that these changes in your dose of hormones are handled by your doctor in sequence rather than in parallel.

CONTROLLING THE SIDE-EFFECTS OF HRT

If you experience side-effects while you are taking HRT (see pp. 52–54), there are several ways that you and your doctor can bring them under control. With time and patience you can adapt your regime by changing the type of hormones, the dose, the route of administration or the medication regime.

Oestrogens can be divided into synthetic types, such as mestranol and ethinyl oestradiol, and natural types like conjugated equine oestrogens and oestradiol varieties. Synthetic oestrogens in higher dosages than those normally used in HRT may increase the risk of thromboembolism (potentially fatal blood clot). Natural oestrogens are usually prescribed in HRT, but you should find out which of these two types you are taking and suggest to your doctor that you switch from a synthetic hormone to a natural one, or, if you are already taking a natural oestrogen, that you try a different brand.

The main progestogens used in HRT vary quite markedly in their effects, and if you have side-effects, lowering the dose or switching to another type of progestogen may help. A drug called tibolone (see p. 49) has few progestogenic side-effects. You can also take your progestogen as suppositories or in gel form; both are good because side-effects are minimal.

TAKING HRT

Most doctors start women off on HRT tablets, but this method does not suit all women. For example, high oral oestrogen can cause nausea (taking your tablet at night may mean that you can sleep through any nausea).

As with any drug taken by mouth (rather than being absorbed through the skin or implanted in the fat layer), a large dose is given because after absorption much of the drug is removed from the bloodstream by the liver. The tablet form of HRT therefore contains more hormone than is necessary to alleviate symptoms and this may explain why you experience side-effects.

If you cut your dosage of oral medication and you still have problems, try switching to a patch form of HRT (see p. 56), which contains much less hormone than oral

HRT, or ask your doctor about an implant, which is formulated to release oestrogen slowly and consistently over a period of four to six months.

If you find that your menopausal symptoms affect your urogenital tract more than any other part of your body, and you have symptoms such as a dry vagina, pain during sex and frequent, urgent urination, then vaginal pessaries or cream may be sufficient to relieve your symptoms. Because these are applied locally, they prevent your whole body from being exposed to hormones. However, creams and pessaries still have the protective qualities of oral HRT on your heart and bones.

Some women who experience progestogenic side-effects such as mood changes respond well to progesterone taken in a suppository form. This may be advantageous in that suppositories contain natural progesterone instead of its synthetic counterpart, progestogen. Some women find that they can tolerate the natural hormone better than synthetic progestogen. However, bigger doses of natural progesterone are needed to control the HRT cycle than if synthetic progestogens are used (this is why progesterone is not widely prescribed). A combination of an oestrogen skin patch and a progesterone suppository may be the best way for you to take HRT.

CHANGING YOUR REGIME

Most women will take continuous oestrogen and 10–14 days of progestogen a month. However, there are several variations in how HRT can be taken, one of which is sure to suit you. If you are taking oestrogen tablets you can begin to leave a space between medications. With your doctor's supervision, you could try taking your tablet two days out of three, three days out of four, or every other day, and see how you feel. Skin patches can be left on for four days at a time instead of three to four, or they can be left off for a day. This may be particularly helpful in relieving mastalgia (breast pain) and weight gain.

You could ask your doctor if you can try the very latest regime, "combined continuous HRT", on which you'll stop bleeding in a few months (see p. 57). If you have progestogenic side-effects and you are taking HRT in which progestogen and oestrogen are combined, ask your doctor to prescribe different products in which the hormones are separate. For example, you could take

INDIVIDUAL TREATMENT

The essence of success in HRT is matching the treatment to each individual woman.

You and your doctor should work together to find the hormone combination that suits you best. In a survey of 100 women, it was found that only 17 percent had stayed on their first treatment over many years, and all the others had made one or two adjustments. If something does not seem right, discuss with your doctor whether the dose or the method is suitable for you. If you're experiencing premenstrual symptoms or have troublesome bleeding, modification of the progestogen may help.

MAXIMIZING INTERNAL OESTROGEN

To compensate for the low levels of oestrogen in your bloodstream, you can boost your own internal oestrogen production in two ways.

The first is exercise, which can be almost as good as HRT in the postmenopausal years when your body needs relatively little oestrogen to thrive.

Your second source of internal oestrogen comes from fat cells, which is why it is dangerous for peri- and postmenopausal women to diet excessively and become underweight. Thin women generally have an earlier menopause than those who are overweight, because fat cells all over your body manufacture oestrogen, and in their absence hormone levels can fall very low.

If you don't wish to take HRT, but are having symptoms of oestrogen deficiency, make sure that you keep your weight up slightly. Whatever you do, don't lose so much weight that you are left with very little body fat, since you will be depriving yourself of an important source of natural oestrogen.

oestrogen in a skin patch form and progestogen in tablet form. This way you and your doctor can juggle the dose of the progestogen so that you have a withdrawal bleed without troublesome side-effects.

FINDING THE RIGHT DOSE

Many people believe that if something is doing you good, taking more will be even better for you. This is not a maxim to which doctors subscribe. As a general principle, doctors prefer you to take the lowest possible dose of any medication for the maximum effect and for the fewest side-effects. As a rule of thumb, medication should be taken for the shortest possible time – HRT is a rare exception to this rule.

It may take a little time to find your optimum dose, and you and your doctor may have to experiment a little because there is no way of anticipating how each individual woman will respond to the many different oestrogens that are available. When you begin to take HRT, it is wise to have a minimum of a four-month trial because it takes that long for your body to settle down. If necessary, your doctor can assess whether your hormone dose is correct by measuring the amount of oestrogen in your bloodstream. Even in low doses, hormones are powerful substances and it is unwise to change your dose without consulting your doctor first.

MONITORING HRT

As you approach the menopause you should be seeing your doctor for annual blood pressure checks, regular cervical smear tests and mammography. Your doctor should also check your weight and carry out a pelvic and breast examination before you take HRT. Once you're taking hormones, you should have these examinations annually, and your weight and blood pressure should be checked every six months. Bone density scans to check on the health of your bones may also be appropriate.

SIDE-EFFECTS AND RISKS

Women are much more likely to give up HRT if their doctors have given them insufficient information. Those who are given a sympathetic hearing and have the opportunity to discuss side-effects have a more realistic view of HRT and tolerate minor side-effects.

The main reasons why women give up HRT are the side-effects of progestogen, the inconvenience of monthly bleeds and a fear of breast cancer. As far as the latter is concerned, the consensus of medical opinion is that there is a very small increase in risk after taking HRT for five years – the same risk as leaving your first baby until you're over 30.

For about 10–15 percent of women, the progestogen is what's so troublesome. To varying degrees, women complain of symptoms such as weight gain, fluid retention, abdominal cramps, backache, acne, greasy skin, irritability, aggressiveness, moodiness, tearfulness and loss of libido. Your doctor can prescribe an alternative form of progestogen or a smaller dose of the one you're taking to alleviate symptoms.

Hypertension (high blood pressure) As hypertension is known to increase the risk of heart attack and strokes, it is a condition that should be taken very seriously in postmenopausal women. Oestrogen will not alter your blood pressure unless you are specifically sensitive to it, which is a very rare phenomenon. This means that you can take HRT even if you do have raised blood pressure, but you should make sure that your blood pressure is checked shortly after starting HRT. If the reading is high, switch from tablets to the patch and speak to your doctor about lifestyle changes that can help, such as diet and exercise.

Breast pain HRT may cause the type of breast swelling and tenderness that is characteristic of the week prior to menstruation. In the first half of the month, the oestrogen in HRT stimulates growth of milk glands and ducts. In the second half of the cycle the progestogen may cause fluid retention within the breast. At this point, the breast may feel as though it is full of orange pips – these are swollen milk glands.

Breast swelling and tenderness may lessen if you cut down your intake of salt, coffee and chocolate, which will also benefit your general health. Taking 100 mg of vitamin B[6] daily for up to five days can also reduce breast pain, and modifying the progestogen dose may help. Breast pain that occurs throughout the HRT cycle is usually due to a dose of oestrogen that is too high.

IRREGULAR BLEEDING

Occasionally, HRT can lead to irregular bleeding, and your doctor will need to take a sample of the uterine lining during hysteroscopy (see p.54) to check and make sure that there are no abnormalities.

You may consider hysteroscopy an inconvenient procedure, but it is best to have an early examination to clear up any possible medical complaints.

HYSTEROSCOPY

This procedure involves examining the inside of the uterus with a small telescopic camera that is passed through the cervix.

Hysteroscopy can be performed under a general anaesthetic, when it may be combined with a dilatation and curettage (D&C), or in the outpatient clinic. If performed as an outpatient procedure, a local anaesthetic may be injected in and around the cervix to help relieve any discomfort. To give a good view, the uterus is distended using a harmless gas such as carbon dioxide, or a liquid.

Most women go home the day of the procedure. For a few days afterwards you may notice some spotting. Some women may need to stay in hospital for a few days if the hysteroscopy has been combined with another operative procedure.

Make sure that you understand why the hysteroscopy is being performed and what is going to be achieved. Hysteroscopy is best avoided if you are pregnant or you are suffering from pelvic inflammatory disease.

Fibroids Benign lumps in the uterine lining may become more widespread if you take HRT and may cause heavy bleeding. However, if your menopausal symptoms are severe, fibroids should not deter you from taking HRT. Any woman with fibroids should have them monitored.

Diabetes If you are diabetic, it's essential to discuss your health with your doctor before embarking on a course of HRT. This is because carbohydrate metabolism is altered by HRT. If you are prescribed HRT, you should check your blood sugar and urine frequently.

Gallstones Between the ages of 50 and 75, three women in 100,000 are estimated to die from complications of gallbladder disease. This rises to six in 100,000 among women taking HRT because oestrogen therapy increases the concentration of the bile in the gallbladder. Obesity is also associated with an increase in gallbladder disease and so it is important to reduce the amount of cholesterol in your diet and to take HRT in a form that does not pass through the liver. The skin patch will be better than a tablet at reducing the possibility of gallstones.

Migraine The response of migraine to HRT is unpredictable. Some women find that their migraines disappear completely while others experience worse attacks. The usual complaint is that migraines occur during the progestogen phase or just after the progestogen is completed. These migraines can often be alleviated by changing the type or dose of progestogen. Migraines at other times in the cycle may be due to low oestrogen levels.

Cancer The possible link between HRT and uterine and breast cancer is a major concern to women. There does appear to be a small increase in the risk of breast cancer after taking HRT for five years. However, the debate surrounding HRT and breast cancer is complicated, since experts do not agree. We now know that the use of progestogen reduces the risk of uterine cancer and may give protection. A persuasive body of evidence shows that in almost all cases of breast disease, HRT is not the cause. If you are not obese, you don't smoke and breast cancer does not run in your family, then the evidence seems to weigh in favour of taking HRT.

TYPES OF MEDICATION

A combined form is the usual way for women with an intact uterus to take HRT; this means that you take both oestrogen and progestogen. Doctors often prescribe these two hormones in tablet form, so that you take oestrogen every day, and progestogen for around 12 days in each month or cycle. The latter induces a withdrawal bleed. However, there are many other ways for you to take oestrogen and progestogen. For example, your doctor may instead prescribe a patch, an implant, a vaginal ring containing oestrogen or an oestrogen cream or gel, or may fit an IUS (an IUD that delivers progestogen or progesterone directly to the uterus) and give oral oestrogen. These many different forms of HRT are known as routes of administration, and each one has its own advantages and disadvantages (see chart, p. 56). They are all very effective at relieving menopausal symptoms, with the exception of oestrogen creams and pessaries, which treat only local urogenital symptoms, for example dryness, soreness or itchiness. These will not help symptoms such as hot flushes or night sweats, but they will still help to prevent a decline in bone density, as some of the other routes of administration can.

The skin patch contains a reservoir of oestrogen that is released transdermally (across the skin) into the body. This means that, unlike HRT taken in tablet form, hormones do not have to pass through the liver – this is advantageous for some women (see Gallstones, p. 54). You may be prescribed progestogen tablets with your patch, or you may be prescribed a combined patch that already contains progestogen. Patches need to be changed every three or four days.

Oestrogen implants also avoid oestrogen having to pass through the liver and once they are inserted by a doctor into the fatty tissue underneath the skin of the abdomen or buttock, they last for up to six months. Progestogen tablets are prescribed with this particular form of oestrogen therapy.

Pessaries and creams
These forms of HRT deliver oestrogen directly into the vagina but the low dose does not offer protection against heart disease or osteoporosis.

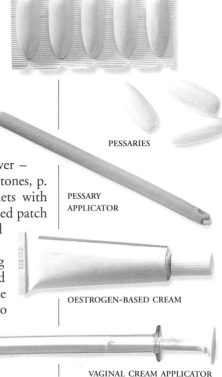

PESSARIES

PESSARY APPLICATOR

OESTROGEN-BASED CREAM

VAGINAL CREAM APPLICATOR

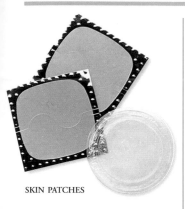

SKIN PATCHES

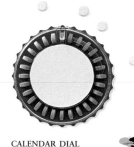

CALENDAR DIAL
OF OESTROGEN

APPLICATOR AND
PHIAL CONTAINING
OESTROGEN PELLET
FOR IMPLANT

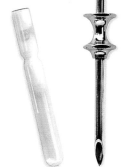

Patches, pills and implants
These forms of HRT deliver
oestrogen directly into the
body. They protect against
osteoporosis and heart
disease and effectively treat
most menopausal symptoms.

TYPES OF HORMONE REPLACEMENT THERAPY

TYPE	ADVANTAGES	DISADVANTAGES
Tablets	• Highly effective in combating physical and emotional symptoms. • Contain oestrogen and/or progestogen. Protect against osteoporosis.	• If does is incorrect you may experience side-effects such as breast tenderness. • You may experience breakthrough bleeding if you forget to take a tablet.
Creams and pessaries	• Help to alleviate urinary incontinence. • Relieve vaginal dryness and itchiness.	• Do not protect against osteoporosis. • Do not combat hot flushes and night sweats. • If used long-term, should be low-dose.
Skin patches or gel	• Equally effective as oral HRT in treating most menopausal symptoms, and preserves bone density in 85–95 percent of women. • Easily changed and simple to stop using.	• A very few women develop red, itchy skin at the site of the patch. This may get worse in a hot climate. • As for tablets, above.
Implants	• Excellent relief from physical symptoms. Protects against osteoporosis. Some women find that problems, such as depression and irritability, disappear more readily than with other forms of HRT. • You can forget you are on HRT. • Testosterone can also be given as an implant.	• Implants are inserted under the skin by your doctor. • Wrong doses cannot be easily modified. • If you decide to stop using HRT, implants are difficult to remove.

TAKING HRT

The three main ways in which HRT medication can be administered are described in the regimes below. The main difference is in the bleeding pattern that results.

Continuous therapy Continuous oestrogen therapy with added progestogen medication has now become the most common way to take HRT. You can take a daily tablet of oestrogen or wear a skin patch twice a week. Progestogen is taken either in pill form or in a combination skin patch for 12–14 days. Over 90 percent of women will have a monthly bleed on this regime if the uterus is intact. Take notice of your bleeding pattern, which should occur after you stop taking progestogen. If bleeding begins before this, the dose of progestogen may be too low for you and should be adjusted.

Cyclical therapy A less common HRT regime is to take oestrogen and progestogen cyclically. Oestrogen is taken from the first day of the cycle to the 21st, and progestogen is added for the last 12 or 13 days of the cycle. Both medications are stopped on the 21st day and a withdrawal bleed will occur between days 22 and 28; the patch- or pill-free days. Over 90 percent of women who have not had a hysterectomy will experience a withdrawal bleed in the interval between ending one treatment and beginning the next. However, bleeding usually lessens over time and may disappear altogether.

The most up-to-date way to take cyclical therapy is to take progestogen once every three months. This means that you go two months without a bleed, then bleed in the third month, so that you have four menstrual periods a year (see p. 49). To find out if this regime is suitable for you, have a chat with your gynaecologist.

Combined continuous therapy (No-bleed HRT) This method of taking HRT involves taking continuous daily doses of both oestrogen and progestogen. The aim of this continuous therapy is to avoid periods, and even if you do have withdrawal bleeding at first, it will probably stop within a few months. No-bleed HRT is popular among women on long-term treatment. Between 50 and 70 percent of women find this regime successful.

IUS

Women who do not wish to bleed and find continuous progestogen by mouth unsatisfactory can have an IUD impregnated with progestogen, known as an IUS, inserted.

Progestogen is released in tiny amounts sufficient to prevent thickening of the endometrium, but the effects are entirely local and therefore unwanted side-effects are minimal. Oestrogen is taken continuously by mouth or via a skin patch.

CONTRA-INDICATIONS

If you have experienced any of the conditions listed below, see the chart on page 59 to identify whether or not HRT is right for you.

- *Any type of abnormal vaginal bleeding.*

- *Breast cancer.*

- *Ovarian cancer.*

- *Uterine cancer.*

- *Recent stroke.*

- *Pancreatic disease.*

- *Recent heart attack.*

- *Recent liver disease.*

- *Recent venous thrombosis (clot in the veins).*

- *Recent pulmonary embolus (clot in the lung).*

- *Uncontrolled high blood pressure.*

- *Undiagnosed breast lump.*

WHEN HRT MAY NOT BE THE ANSWER

The term "contraindication" refers to a medical condition that may be exacerbated by a particular drug. In the case of HRT, it was once thought that some conditions were "absolute contraindications", such as breast cancer or uterine cancer. However, some doctors now believe that there is no such thing as an absolute contraindication, and that only "relative" contraindications exist, provided that the dose and route of administration is individually tailored. Other doctors subscribe to the theory that certain medical conditions (see left) make it risky to take HRT. The items in this list are still frequently quoted as contraindications, but when they are scrutinized, the dangers diminish (and in some instances disappear). This is partly because of increased medical understanding, but mainly because theoretical disadvantages of HRT can be overcome by careful adjustments to therapy and tailoring the HRT regime to suit each patient.

In older lists of this kind, angina and a family history of heart attacks, strokes and venous thrombosis may have been included. Now, these conditions are regarded as positive indications for HRT, since HRT may protect you against them.

CONTRAINDICATIONS IN PERSPECTIVE

The first warnings about contraindications were based on the oral contraceptive pill (which contains a much higher dose of hormones than HRT), and they are therefore not directly referable to HRT. Lists of contraindications for HRT are usually supplied by drug companies who have special reasons (for example avoidance of litigation) for including a wide range of conditions that do not necessarily reflect medical thinking or practice.

You need to evaluate the pros and cons of taking HRT. Although it treats your menopausal symptoms, if you have had a condition such as breast cancer your doctor may be reluctant to prescribe HRT. These decisions should be negotiable. If you can't cope with hot flushes and night sweats, and your doctor is unsympathetic, go to a gynaecologist or a menopause clinic who may try to find a suitable form of HRT for you.

HRT AND YOUR MEDICAL HISTORY

Do you have, or have you ever had, any of the following?	Can you take HRT if you have, or have had, this condition?	Take note of these comments that reflect the latest thinking of experts in the field of HRT·
Unexplained abnormal vaginal bleeding	No	Any unusual bleeding must be thoroughly investigated by your doctor.
Breast cancer	Possibly not. Must be discussed fully with your doctor.	Prescribing HRT to women with these conditions is very controversial, but some doctors and gynaecologists believe that as long as the form and dose of HRT is carefully chosen, HRT is safe.
Ovarian cancer		
Uterine cancer		
Stroke		
Pancreatic disease		
Angina	Yes	
Gallstones	Yes	
Heart attack	Yes	If you have had a recent heart attack you should not take HRT. However, if you have had a heart attack in the past then you can take HRT, provided you have three-monthly cardiovascular tests.
Liver disease	Yes	If you have had liver disease in the past you can take HRT. If a liver function test is abnormal at any time you should avoid HRT.
Deep vein thrombosis	No	If you have had a thrombosis, you should not take HRT.
Pulmonary embolus	No	If you have had a pulmonary embolism, you should not take HRT.
Diabetes mellitus	Yes	Have your blood sugar and urine checked frequently.
Corticosteroid therapy	Yes	Corticosteroids (which are used to treat rheumatoid arthritis) have a detrimental effect on bone health. Taking HRT will compensate.
Ovarian cysts, fibroids, endometriosis, migraine	Yes	Use the skin patch method of HRT.
Varicose veins	Yes	If your veins become inflamed, consult your doctor.

SERMS

SERMS are a class of drug called Selective oEstrogen Receptor Modulators that can be used for the prevention of vertebral fractures in postmenopausal women who are at increased risk of developing osteoporosis.

Clinical trials also show that SERMS reduce total and LDL (unhealthy) cholesterol levels and so protect against heart disease. In preliminary clinical trials they reduced the frequency of newly diagnosed breast cancer by more than 50 percent in women taking the drug for two years or more.

In some parts of the body SERMS act like oestrogen, but in others they don't. Through their selective action they provide women with the benefit of oestrogen on bones and the heart while blocking oestrogen's effect on the breast and uterus. However, SERMS do not treat menopausal symptoms such as hot flushes and vaginal dryness, nor do they protect against the onset of Alzheimer's disease as HRT does.

SERMS is taken as a once-daily tablet and is intended for long-term use. As with most drugs, SERMS do have some side-effects, most of which are mild. They include hot flushes and leg cramps, but these are not usually serious enough to stop taking the drug. SERMS therapy also has a small increased risk of venous thrombosis (less than 1 percent).

IT'S NEVER TOO LATE TO START

A woman is never too old to start taking HRT, either for menopausal symptoms, which don't necessarily decline when periods cease and may re-emerge during their 60s and 70s, and for purely medical reasons when HRT can be life-saving.

More than a few women experience hot flushes and night sweats that are troublesome enough to merit treatment for the first time in their middle 60s and even later or after having stopped HRT. I receive hundreds of letters from these women who find that their doctors are reluctant to treat them with HRT and who say that the symptoms aren't related to the menopause. They are wrong. We know that the symptoms are menopausal and respond well to HRT. An older woman whose doctor won't prescribe HRT should ask for a referral to a gynaecologist who certainly will.

There are many medical reasons for prescribing HRT, in addition to helping classical menopausal symptoms. Talk to your doctor about whether or not HRT is advisable for you. Symptoms of osteoporosis, such as severe bone pain, decrease in height, collapsed vertebrae or fracture, are strong reasons for taking HRT because it can rebuild bone to its former strength in little more than two years and so will prevent further problems. A recent US study of long-term HRT use has shown a 34 percent reduction in hip fractures and a 24 percent reduction in overall fractures in menopausal women. If you have brittle bones, you may be advised to stay on HRT for life.

If you're a high-risk woman for osteoporosis or bowel cancer you're a candidate for starting HRT at the menopause to lower your risk. HRT has been shown to lower a menopausal woman's risk of a bowel cancer by 37 percent, so if you have a family history of bowel cancer or have taken steroids, you should take HRT early for your health's sake. It's never too late to start taking HRT and there's no age when you need to stop taking it. Indeed there's no reason to stop taking HRT at all, if you don't want to.

HEALTH CHECKS

Monitoring your health is the key to continuing a
healthy and active life. Observing and reading the
messages your body sends, then responding to them,
brings a great sense of satisfaction and well-being.
Being aware of your health gives you control over
your body, and helps you to spot potential medical
conditions early, when they may be more easily and
successfully treated. Far and away the most
important health checks for menopausal women are
breast self-examination and mammography – which
you should have at least every two years.

MEDICAL TESTS

Doctors can monitor your physical health during the menopause with a range of medical procedures. Here are the most common ones.

- *Eye test.*

- *Blood test for hormone levels and thyroid function.*

- *Mammogram.*

- *Blood pressure test.*

- *Blood test for high cholesterol.*

- *Urine test for diabetes.*

- *Cervical smear test.*

- *Bone density scan.*

- *Electrocardiogram.*

MONITORING YOUR HEALTH

As you reach the menopause you will need to have a variety of health checks done regularly. Certain tests that you have had in the past will be carried out more frequently, while new tests may need to be done because of your changed status as a menopausal woman. There are also procedures such as colposcopy (see p. 67) that may need to be done if routine checks reveal any abnormalities. Ideally, there will be a large team of people to help monitor your health, of whom you are the first member. The others would include your doctor and gynaecologist, the radiologist who interprets your mammogram, the cytologist who reads your smear and so on. Think of them as a supportive team with whom you can interact, discuss and make informed decisions.

Doctors have a responsibility to women on hormone replacement therapy (see HRT, pp. 43–60), and, before HRT is prescribed, your doctor should carry out an examination of your breasts, take a cervical smear and check your weight and blood pressure. Ideally, you should have a mammogram to assess the health of your breasts and a bone density test to predict your likelihood of developing osteoporosis. Once you are taking HRT, you should have annual consultations with your doctor in which you discuss any side-effects and bleeding, and have your weight and blood pressure checked.

SELF-CHECKS

There are several checks you can do to monitor your health. For example, excess weight at 55 is much more difficult to lose than at 35, so it's worth keeping a weekly check on your weight. This way you should never have more than a few kilograms or pounds to shed and can take immediate steps to lose them over a few weeks.

You can also assess what stage of the menopause you have reached by keeping a detailed diary of your menstrual periods, physical symptoms and mood changes. This information will lead to increased self-awareness and may help you to develop strategies, including taking HRT, to cope with menopausal symptoms.

BREASTS

In some women the menopause can bring with it an enormous increase in the size of the breasts, and they may be tender and even painful. A possible explanation for this is the increase with age of menstrual cycles in which we don't ovulate (see p. 15). This means that there is no progesterone to control the effect of oestrogen. The breasts are therefore exposed to prolonged periods of unopposed oestrogen stimulation and swell as a result.

BREAST SELF-EXAMINATION

It is important to examine your breasts once a month. If you are still menstruating, the best time is at the end of your period when your breasts are not swollen or tender. You can do a breast examination at any time of the month if you are postmenopausal.

How to feel your breasts
Lie on your back with your head on a pillow and your shoulders slightly raised. Keep the arm you are not using by your side and with your fingers flat, examine each section of the breast using gentle circular movements. Finish by extending the arm you are not using behind your head and checking for lumps along the collar bone and in your armpits.

Check for swollen lymph nodes in your armpits

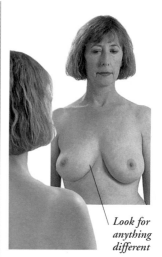

Look for anything different

What to look for
Stand naked in front of a mirror. Observe your breasts with your arms at your sides, then raised with your hands behind your head. Look for differences in the shape or texture of your breasts and nipples, and for swellings or lumps, a dimpled, puckered appearance or a newly inverted nipple.

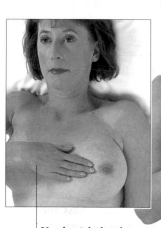

Use the right hand to feel the left breast and vice versa

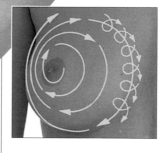

Feeling pattern
Move your hand in towards the nipple, using a clockwise circular direction on the left breast and an anti-clockwise direction on the right breast.

RECOMMENDED TIMING

If you have not had a mammogram performed in the last year, and you are planning to take HRT, your doctor may suggest you have one done before you start treatment. Every time you ask for your HRT prescription to be repeated, you can ask your doctor to perform a manual examination of your breasts in addition to the one you carry out yourself.

If your mammogram reveals a lump you will probably be advised not to take HRT until the cause of the lump has been diagnosed. This is because some doctors regard breast cancer as a reason not to take HRT. However, some gynaecologists will tailor the dose and method of giving you HRT to suit your individual needs, placing you at minimal risk.

MAMMOGRAPHY

This is a type of X-ray, known as a "soft" X-ray, that reveals changes in the consistency of breast tissue, including cysts and tumours. Mammograms penetrate only a few centimetres and are harmless. A radiologist uses them to locate any areas of increased density in the breast, possibly even calcification, which may indicate abnormalities or cancer.

HOW IS A MAMMOGRAM DONE?

To have a mammogram, you will need to be naked from the waist upwards and stand in different positions so that your breasts can be X-rayed from various angles. In order to photograph every angle, the breasts may sometimes have to be gently compressed between two X-ray plates; although you may find this uncomfortable, it is not usually painful, unless your breasts are tender.

Mammography is a particularly reliable technique for the examination of large breasts, since accurate pictures are obtained and there is a high degree of contrast between normal tissue and abnormal structures. A radiologist will be able to use a mammogram to discern extremely small cysts and tiny tumours that you would not be able to feel or notice yourself during your monthly breast examination.

Mammograms are likely to be less revealing if you have had breast implants, since these can obscure the view of the breast tissue. Mammograms also tend to be less accurate on small-breasted women.

FREQUENCY OF PROCEDURE

You should have a mammogram every two years from the age of 45, or earlier if you have a family history of breast cancer, particularly if your mother or sister had the disease. Because mammography can detect minute tumours before they have the chance to spread, it is the most important procedure for the early detection of breast cancer. Research data shows that almost 90 percent of breast cancers detected by mammography emerge in the first "baseline" reading. If your baseline reading is clear, it is less likely that any tumours will be found in subsequent mammograms. The procedure will, however, show up any later changes.

BONE DENSITY

In the first few years after oestrogen levels decline, many women go through a phase of rapid bone density loss. Oestrogen is crucial in maintaining bone repair, a process called remodelling, and without sufficient oestrogen you lose more bone than you build up, resulting in fragile bones and osteoporosis (see pp. 70–76). Within a few years of the menopause, the rate of bone loss slows down, but by that time, the damage could be irreparable.

BONE DENSITY SCANS

A bone density scan provides a window on your skeleton. It's based on the principle that X-rays cannot penetrate hard structures such as bone; the whiter your bone X-rays are, the more dense and healthy your bone. The darker the X-ray, the less dense your bones are, and the more brittle they are likely to be.

A bone density scan is useful both as a diagnostic tool, to reveal osteoporosis for the first time, and as a way of monitoring progress after treatment for osteoporosis has begun. Experts in this field suggest that one bone density measurement around the time of the menopause can predict your future risk of osteoporotic fractures. Women can be divided into two risk groups: those with low bone mass and high risk of future fracture, and those with high bone mass and low risk of fracture.

HOW IS THE SCAN DONE?

Dual energy X-ray absorptiometry (DEXA) is currently the most precise and widely used method of assessing bone density. This non-invasive procedure can be carried out in hospital X-ray departments, menopause clinics, well-woman clinics and consultants' surgeries. Your bone density is assessed by a radiologist.

To have the scan, you lie on a table and a radiation beam is passed over you. The density of the spine and the thigh bone usually provide a good indication of bone health throughout the body. In a similar technique, called single photon absorptiometry, the bones in your wrist are measured. You place your arm between a beam of low-level radiation and a detector. Your X-rays will be rated on a specially devised scale, which correlates the appearance of bone X-rays with bone health.

WHO NEEDS A BONE DENSITY SCAN?

In my opinion, all women with menopausal symptoms, but particularly those suffering from bone, muscle, back and joint pain, should have a bone density scan.

The best time to have the scan done is when your symptoms first start, but any time during the menopause is sufficient.

*Recent experimental research
has revealed that the presence
of a hormone called inhibin
may be a forewarning of
ovarian cancer.*

*Inhibin can be identified with
a simple blood test, which is a
more straightforward and less
traumatic procedure than a
laparoscopy (inserting a tube
through the abdominal wall).*

*Inhibin appears very early in
the course of the disease – as
much as 20 months before the
actual cancer shows – making
early diagnosis possible. This is
a potentially great advance in
the management of ovarian
cancer, because tumours can
grow quite large and spread
before they cause symptoms.*

*Cure rates are directly related
to early diagnosis, so this test
could increase survival rates
significantly. Monitoring
inhibin levels also reveals
whether treatment is working,
but this test is likely to be
available at only a few
specialized centres.*

TESTS ON THE UTERUS AND OVARIES

Between the ages of 55 and 65, the incidence of uterine cancer more than doubles. Malignant ovarian growths are also most common after the age of 50.

CERVICAL SMEAR TEST

Although cervical cancer is comparatively rare in postmenopausal women, the cervical smear test is so effective in the prevention of cervical cancer it is an important gynaecological test for women of all ages. Before cancer develops there is a precancerous stage that is symptomless and does not produce signs that are visible to the naked eye. However, there are cellular changes in the cervix and by taking a sample of cervical cells, staining them and examining them under a microscope, doctors can identify any abnormalities and decide upon the appropriate treatment.

If abnormal cervical cells are discovered as the result of a smear test, the changes are classified as mild, moderate or severe (see Test Results, right). In the first case, a repeat smear test will be recommended in three to six months' time, since sometimes abnormalities can simply disappear. If the cell changes are moderate or severe, a procedure known as a colposcopy (see right), which allows your doctor to see a microscopic level of detail on your cervix, is likely to be recommended. Occasionally, women may be called back for a repeat smear – not because there are any abnormalities, but because the smear is "unreadable". This may be because either blood or inflammatory cells were present (you should not have a smear test while you are menstruating or if you have a gynaecological infection), or because the cells were collected from the wrong part of the cervix.

The area of the cervix that is affected by abnormal cell growth is called the transformation zone, and its exact location depends on a woman's age. In postmenopausal women the transformation zone moves up into the cervical canal, making the zone less accessible during a smear test. This is remedied by the use of an endocervical brush, which can be gently inserted into the cervical canal to gather the sample of cells.

A common reason for abnormal changes in the cervix is the genital wart or human papilloma virus (HPV). Some types of HPV can cause changes that show up in a smear test, but as many as a third of these abnormalities can disappear spontaneously. For this reason, if you have a history of genital warts, you should make sure that you have a smear test every two or three years. Other women should have a smear test every five years.

HOW IS A CERVICAL SMEAR DONE?

A smear test entails an internal examination in which a speculum is inserted into the vagina. The speculum holds open the vagina and allows your doctor to gain access to the cervix and note any abnormal changes. A thin layer of cells from the cervix and some mucus are collected. A smear test is carried out when you are lying down with your knees apart. Although you may feel a mild scraping sensation, the procedure should be painless.

TEST RESULTS AND RECOMMENDATIONS

The results of a smear test are classified into four or five categories. Negative gives you the all-clear; no follow-up is needed. Your next smear should be in three years' time. The mildest inflammation is known as mild dysplasia (called CIN I); this means you have some infection and should be tested again in six months' time. A positive smear test means there is a detectable change in the cells necessitating further investigation. For moderate dysplasia (called CIN II), this will be a colposcopy; for severe dysplasia with or without invasive cancer (called CIN III), this will be a colposcopy with or without cone biopsy (see column, right).

COLPOSCOPY

If a smear test reveals any abnormal cells, this is a further non-invasive procedure that a specialist will use to decide on an appropriate treatment. Using apparatus resembling a pair of binoculars on a stand, a microscopic level of detail can be seen on the surface of the cervix. Expert colposcopists can recognize chronic inflammation, infection, polyps and areas of pre-invasive cancer. If your colposcopist finds something that appears abnormal to the eye, he or she may recommend laser treatment, a cone biopsy or loop excision (see column, right).

CONE BIOPSY

This procedure is done if a colposcopy (see left) shows the presence of cancerous cells in the cervix, or if a colposcopy is inconclusive. The latter is likely to be the case for women over 35, because less of their cervical tissue can be seen due to retraction of the cervix caused by age.

Under general anaesthetic, a piece of the cervix in the shape of a cone is removed using a laser or scalpel. The base of the cone is on the outside of the cervix and the apex is deep in the cervical tissue. This cone is then finely dissected so that the exact extent of disease can be determined. The area will be stitched to reduce bleeding, although diathermy (electrical stimulation) or freezing is also effective as an alternative.

LOOP EXCISION

The most recent procedure for removing abnormal cervical cells is loop excision.

This straightforward technique involves the removal of tissue using a heated wire loop. Its great advantage is that it can be performed in the outpatient department of a hospital without the need for a general anaesthetic. Loop excision also removes a smaller amount of tissue than a cone biopsy.

CARDIOVASCULAR (HEART) TESTS

If you have no symptoms, you exercise several times a week, you are not overweight and don't smoke, it's very unlikely that you have any heart disease, and occasional check-ups will be sufficient.

Heart checks include listening to your heart, measuring your blood pressure, and possibly having an electrocardiogram (ECG) and a blood test. If you have raised blood pressure or high blood cholesterol, a family history of heart disease, you are overweight, you smoke or you rarely exercise, you should have annual heart check-ups from the age of 35. You should not need an ECG unless your doctor finds an abnormality.

An ECG can be done in a doctor's office, at home or in a hospital. Electrodes connected to a recording machine are applied to your chest, wrists and ankles. Electrical signals, which record the contractions of the heart muscle, are charted and displayed as a trace on a moving graph or screen. To an expert, this reveals detailed information about the health and functioning of your heart. Minute changes on the tracing reflect potentially dangerous changes in your heart function.

In conjunction with an ECG, you may be given an exercise tolerance test. You will be asked to perform a set exercise, such as walking on a motorized treadmill, and a reading will be taken to record your heart's response to the extra strain.

OTHER TESTS

With the first symptom of the menopause, your doctor may suggest checking on your level of oestrogen and, since heart disease is the greatest killer of postmenopausal women, checking your heart, too.

HORMONE LEVEL TEST

Specialized hormone tests are more likely to be carried out by gynaecologists than by doctors, although you may find that hospital clinics adapt some procedures slightly.

Profound changes happen to your sex hormones at the menopause (and then again in your 70s and 80s). The two major oestrogen hormones, oestradiol and oestrone, plummet after the menopause, and oestradiol stays low for the rest of your life unless HRT is taken. Oestrone follows a slightly different pattern. During a woman's 50s, 60s and 70s, levels decline, but after that oestrone begins to increase. Low levels of oestrone or oestradiol in midlife mean that the menopause is imminent. This shows up in a blood test as high levels of follicle stimulating hormone (FSH) and luteinizing hormone (LH).

If you go to see your doctor when you are symptomless, before the onset of the menopause, it's unlikely that you'll convince him or her of the need to carry out hormone tests. If, however, you have early symptoms of the menopause, such as the occasional hot flush, back pain or slight dryness of the vagina, it could be that you're on the rising part of the curve, and this could easily be confirmed by performing a blood test for FSH or LH.

RECOMMENDATIONS

I feel that information about hormone depletion is crucial for women who are approaching or going through the menopause. It gives you knowledge about what's going on internally, which can help you to understand the symptoms that you may be experiencing. It also means you can plan ways of dealing with the menopause. For example, you can argue your case for HRT if, having read the table on page 45, you feel you are a candidate for it and would benefit from it. If you have a family history of heart disease or brittle bones, low blood hormone levels of FSH and LH will support the case for your taking HRT before the onset of the menopause.

6

LONG-TERM HEALTH AND HRT

The falling level of oestrogen during the menopause together with the natural ageing process in the postmenopausal years means that women can become increasingly susceptible to illness and disease. One of the most painful conditions is osteoporosis, which is the single most important health hazard for women past the menopause – it is more common than heart disease, stroke, diabetes or breast cancer. Other more minor conditions, for example cystitis, urinary incontinence and pelvic prolapse, are not life-threatening but may still cause women considerable distress. These can be overcome with a combination of preventive, medical and self-help measures.

As oestrogen and progesterone levels fall, bones begin to lose mass by 0.5–3 percent a year. An 80-year-old woman can easily have lost 40 percent of the bone mass in her body.

Healthy bone has blood vessels and nerves and a very efficient system for maintenance and repair. There are special cells called osteoblasts, that renew, repair and lay down new bone. The activity of these cells is controlled mainly by hormones, including oestrogen, which is thought to increase the repair and renewal rate of bone. If oestrogen levels fall, bone is not replaced as efficiently.

Bone that is healthy is rich in calcium. Oestrogen facilitates the uptake of calcium from the blood into the bone and inhibits calcium loss. A fall in oestrogen levels therefore leads to bone disintegration.

When tiny holes form within the bone, two things happen. First, the overall structure and supporting tissue of the bone is thinned out and, second, there is less of the inner, spongy bone matrix in which calcium can be deposited. Eventually the tiny craters in bone expand to look like holes in Swiss cheese. Bones lose their thickness and density and become brittle and break with relative ease. For a woman with severe osteoporosis of the spine, minor knocks, jolts or falls can cause the spinal bones to fracture.

BRITTLE BONES (OSTEOPOROSIS)

A painful, crippling and life-threatening condition, osteoporosis is the single most important health hazard for women past the menopause – it is more common than heart disease, stroke, diabetes or breast cancer. In its early stages, osteoporosis has no obvious symptoms, so many women may be unaware that they have it. Because of its life-threatening nature, it is vital that all women be told the facts about this disease, and take measures to prevent osteoporosis from destroying their lives.

The word "osteoporosis" is derived from the Greek and means "bone that has many holes". A clinical definition of osteoporosis is "a condition where there is less normal bone than expected for a woman's age, with an increased risk of fracture". However, some experts restrict the term "osteoporosis" to describe low bone density where fractures have already occurred, and use the term "osteopenia" to describe women who have bones with low density, but have not suffered fractures. Osteoporosis is commonly called "brittle bone disease".

RISK FACTORS

Ageing is the main cause of osteoporosis, but it can also be the result of malignant disease, chronic liver disorder or rheumatoid arthritis. Black women, who have greater bone density, have a lower risk of developing osteoporosis than white women. Certain conditions, situations and habits (see pp. 71–72) are also contributory factors. The most significant of these is impaired peak bone density.

LOW BONE DENSITY

From infancy, your bones grow in size until peak bone mass or density is achieved between the ages 25 and 35. After this point bone mass no longer increases. The amount of bone in your skeleton as you approach the menopause will depend on three things: the peak level of bone mass you achieved, the time at which your bone loss begins and the rate at which bone loss proceeds. If your peak bone mass is low to begin with, you have a much greater chance of developing severe osteoporosis after the menopause.

AMENORRHOEA

Osteoporosis occurs in some women with premenopausal amenorrhoea (lack of menstrual periods), and is related to low oestrogen levels. Two examples of high risk categories are young women with anorexia nervosa and young sportswomen who exercise excessively while living on a restricted diet. When the body receives so little food that the fat-to-muscle ratio drops, it responds by switching off oestrogen production in the ovaries.

HYPERTHYROIDISM

Women who have an overactive thyroid gland or who take high doses of thyroxine for thyroid deficiency are at risk of developing osteoporosis. Women overtreated with thyroxine may lose bone mass at seven times the normal rate. If you are taking thyroxine, ask your doctor to check your thyroid function and dosage requirements periodically, and ask about a bone density test.

PREMATURE MENOPAUSE

The earlier the age of the menopause, with its depletion of oestrogen, the greater the risk of osteoporosis. The National Osteoporosis Society (see p. 94) reports that a very high number of women aged between 60 and 69 who have osteoporosis had a premature menopause. While most doctors would offer hormone replacement therapy (see HRT, pp. 43–60) to treat the more obvious and immediate menopausal symptoms, such as hot flushes and night sweats, they often neglect prescribing it for the full length of time needed to protect against osteoporosis.

HYSTERECTOMY AND OVARIAN REMOVAL

The ovaries are a woman's main source of oestrogen, so it is not surprising that their removal leads to loss of bone mass. Most women show early signs of osteoporosis within four years of removal of the ovaries if HRT is not given. Even women who have had hysterectomies without having the ovaries removed are more prone to bone loss than women who retain their uterus.

The National Osteoporosis Society produced statistics showing that only two women out of 100 who had had hysterectomies and removal of the ovaries had been offered HRT, although this situation has improved.

FACTORS AFFECTING PEAK BONE MASS

How much tissue your bones contain when they are at their most dense is the best determinant of how much will be present when you're older. The density of bone is affected by the following:

- *Adequate amounts of both calcium and vitamin D. They are essential for bone health.*

- *Little or no exercise in your 20s will lower peak bone mass; too much exercise, causing amenorrhoea (lack of menstrual periods), is also unhealthy.*

- *The early onset of menstrual periods, a late menopause, taking hormonal contraceptives and multiple pregnancies have a positive effect on bone mass.*

- *Traits inherited from parents. If your parents have thick or heavy bones, generally you will have a similar bone structure.*

"DOWAGER'S" "HUMP"

This debilitating condition has four characteristics: loss of height, hunched posture, a protruding abdomen and a shuffling gait.

As the bones of the spine gradually lose density, the collapse of the vertebrae causes the ribcage to tilt downwards towards the hips. A curvature in the upper spine creates a second curve in the lower spinal column, pushing the internal organs outwards.

Because the spinal column is compressed, up to 20 cm (8 in) in height can be lost. Internal functions are impaired as the compressed organs shift position and obstruct other organs and systems. Constipation can be a problem; breathing may become laboured; and aches and pains in the lower back and throughout the body may arise from pressure on the nerves emanating from the collapsed vertebrae. Managing life day-to-day can become increasingly difficult.

SMOKING

The menopause may start up to five years early in heavy smokers. Smoking severely reduces the benefits of HRT to bone health, and limits the amount of oxygen your body can take in. When oxygen consumption is low, bones tend to be weak. Passive smokers are also at risk. Blood tests have shown that a passive smoker inhales one-fifteenth of the nicotine that is inhaled by a smoker in the same room. Female passive smokers, on average, reach the menopause about three years earlier than women in non-smoking households. The golden rules are to stop smoking well before the menopause and to avoid spending time in a smoke-filled environment.

CORTICOSTEROIDS

Some of the most dangerous drugs that cause bones to become osteoporotic are steroids, such as cortisone or prednisone. These drugs are used to treat many conditions, including severe cases of rheumatoid arthritis and asthma. When prescribed over long periods of time in high doses, corticosteroid usage can lead to osteoporosis. If you are taking these drugs, ask your doctor to prescribe the lowest effective dose, in order to minimize bone damage.

DIAGNOSING OSTEOPOROSIS

Successful treatment and possible prevention of osteoporosis depend on early detection of bone changes. Both sufferers and potential sufferers need to be identified. Your mobility and self-esteem may be severely affected if you allow osteoporosis to progress to the point where it causes severe medical problems, particularly spinal and hip fractures (see right) – a third of women over 65 will suffer a fracture of the spine, and by the age of 90, a third of women will have had a hip fracture. Both can be extremely painful and can make you housebound. These physical problems may be compounded by feelings of awkwardness or a loss in confidence. Take matters into your own hands and make sure you are given the treatments you need to keep your bones strong and healthy.

If you are 50 or over, any curvature of the spine (called kyphosis) and loss of height deserve particular attention. Other common symptoms of osteoporosis include pain, breathlessness, indigestion, acid reflux and urinary incontinence. If you suddenly begin to suffer low-back pain, you should ask your doctor to carry out a test for spinal osteoporosis, and consider the possibility of spinal fracture. No one can tell with complete certainty whether you will develop osteoporosis, although bone density scans (see p. 65), which measure the density of high-risk areas such as the wrist, can provide the most accurate predictions.

FRACTURES

Osteoporosis usually stays undetected in the early stages, and most osteoporotic fractures caused by minor trauma are still not diagnosed as being due to osteoporosis. The working rule is that if you sustain a fracture after minor trauma, osteoporosis is present. Therefore, if you are over 40 and you fracture your wrist or hip after a minor fall, you are likely to have osteoporosis. Fractures of the wrist are known as Colles' fractures and usually result from attempting to break a fall with the hand. Hip fractures are one of the most serious types of fracture, since they are very painful and can severely impair mobility. Compression fractures of the vertebrae are also common, and if you don't receive treatment, you may experience further fractures. Don't leave it too late: 30 percent of your bone mass may have been lost by the time you have a hip fracture.

BACKACHE

Constant pain in the lower back should be taken as a sign for you to seek treatment from a menopause clinic, well-woman clinic, doctor or gynaecologist. (Another common cause of backache in menopausal women is prolapse; see column, p. 89.)

On average, women who develop spinal osteoporosis begin to notice an increase in the occurrence of severe backache about nine to ten years after their final menstrual period, or sooner if they have had a surgically induced menopause (as a result of surgical removal of the ovaries or hysterectomy).

Sufferer may feel housebound

Lack of exercise and vitamin D

Loss of self-esteem

Painful vertebral fractures

Clothes don't fit properly

Pain on movement

Immobility leads to further bone loss and fractures

Fear of being pushed in crowds

The vicious circle of vertebral collapse
Women who suffer from osteoporosis can find themselves trapped in a vicious circle that gradually erodes both their health and their sense of self-esteem.

MEDICAL TREATMENT

The aim of prescription drugs is to halt bone loss, prevent further fractures and replace or repair bone whenever possible. Once fractures occur, at least a third of bone mass has already been lost; in some cases as much as 60 percent is gone.

Over two million people in the UK have already suffered osteoporotic fractures, and although there are some treatments that can reverse osteoporosis, broken joints or bones that have been severely damaged are not likely to respond to treatment. Fortunately, there are several methods that can be effective in halting bone loss, the most potent treatment being HRT.

HORMONE REPLACEMENT THERAPY (HRT)

If you have low bone mass, it is highly recommended that you take HRT. Even if you have high bone mass, your future risk of fracture will be reduced with HRT. Calcium loss can be reduced by taking very low doses of oestrogen, and several studies have suggested that when progestogen (the synthetic version of progesterone) is taken with oestrogen, bone metabolism responds favourably. The progestogen appears to stimulate a small amount of bone formation, while the oestrogen halts further loss of bone.

Studies have also demonstrated that oestrogen therapy helps bone to maintain its mineral strength and mass. With high dosage, oestrogen can increase bone mass in the spine, but a low dose merely slows down the natural ageing loss. Studies show that menopausal women who used oral contraceptives (containing oestrogen) for long periods of time have heavier and stronger bones than women who have never taken oral contraceptives. A new class of drugs known as SERMS (see p.60) can also help to prevent bone loss.

NON-HORMONAL TREATMENT

The first line of defence against osteoporosis is increasing calcium intake through diet. Eat plenty of calcium-rich foods, including dairy products and canned fish with bones, such as sardines, and ask your doctor about calcium supplements. To maximize benefits, calcium should be taken with other treatments, such as HRT.

The drug etidronate has been shown to be effective in treating established spinal osteoporosis. It works by inhibiting the bone-resorbing cells (the osteoclasts) and allowing the bone-rebuilding cells (the osteoblasts) to work more efficiently. This results in a small net gain in the amount of bone in the vertebrae. However, research studies have not yet given us conclusive evidence of etidronate's effectiveness against hip fractures.

Sodium fluoride (available only at specialist treatment centres and not on prescription) can stimulate bone formation and may be given to women with severe vertebral osteoporosis. It is given in daily doses and must be taken with calcium supplements. A low, controlled dose can increase bone density and may reduce fracture rate. However, in higher doses, it can be associated with an increase in hip fractures. Careful monitoring is required when taking sodium fluoride because there may be side-effects of indigestion and nausea.

PAIN RELIEF

Women with vertebral osteoporosis can suffer intense back pain, especially after a new fracture. If pain is very acute, a strong pain-reliever, such as morphine, will be prescribed. This produces rapid relief and may make a journey to hospital more comfortable. Curvature of the spine (called kyphosis) produces ongoing muscular and ligament pain, but this can be treated with painkillers, such as paracetamol or codeine. Paracetamol is a safe, non-addictive drug, although you should be careful not to exceed the recommended dose or frequency of use; codeine may cause constipation.

Physiotherapists may also use various forms of electrotherapy or ultrasound to help relieve pain. Some now also use complementary techniques, for example acupuncture, and recommend the use of heat pads, hot-water bottles or ice packs at home. TENS (Transcutaneous Electrical Nerve Stimulation) machines are available in most treatment centres for pain relief.

If you have back pain, an occupational therapist can advise you on how to organize your home and work environment. You should sit in chairs with high backs that give support to the whole spine, and your bed should be firm, but not so hard that it cannot accommodate the altered shape of your spine.

PHYSIOTHERAPY

Increased muscle strength, improved spinal power and posture, maintenance of bone strength, relief of pain and toning of pelvic floor muscles to cope with stress incontinence are all benefits of physiotherapy.

Special exercises can also help with breathing difficulties that are exacerbated if the head falls forward, causing compression of the chest. Physiotherapy is often overlooked, but it should be an important part of your treatment for osteoporosis. A home exercise programme can be established to continue the treatment.

One of the most basic lessons taught by physiotherapists is how to breathe correctly. You don't need to go to a class to learn, but it is helpful initially to have a teacher's supervision to make sure you are learning the techniques correctly. People who keep themselves supple with exercise and special physiotherapy regimes are less likely to fall over, and they do less damage to themselves when they do fall than people who don't take regular exercise.

Hydrotherapy is another form of physiotherapy. It involves exercising in a pool of water at body temperature, 37°C (98°F), allowing you to move easily while the water supports you. The warmth relaxes the muscles and joints, relieves pain and increases mobility. Buoyancy makes exercise easier, while the water resistance strengthens muscles.

Since the greatest danger of osteoporosis is fracture, it is vital that you help yourself prevent its occurrence.

As women get older, falls can be related to poor coordination and blackouts, so you should ask your doctor to check your heart and blood pressure. It is also important to maintain good vision by having your eyes tested regularly, particularly for a condition known as glaucoma, which becomes more common with age. Avoid sedatives and other drugs that might reduce your alertness, such as antihistamines, and try to limit your alcohol intake.

Reduce hazards at home by removing any trailing electrical flexes and loose carpets. Make sure that stairs have a firm handrail and be particularly on guard when walking on slippery or uneven surfaces.

Many women with painful spinal fractures suffer severe loss of confidence and self-esteem in a vicious circle of physical and emotional distress (see p. 73). In some women, loss of self-esteem may lead to problems that are as serious as their physical discomfort.

Counselling, emotional support from friends and family and talking to other menopausal women with similar problems can do much to give a woman a more positive attitude to life and help her become more outgoing and confident.

PREVENTING OSTEOPOROSIS

Since all of us are at risk of developing osteoporosis, it is important that we adopt self-help measures in order to build up our natural resistance to this life-threatening disease. Fortunately, there are a number of ways in which we can change our lifestyles to help maintain healthy bones. Regular exercise, a balanced diet and mental alertness can help to maintain overall fitness. You should also have regular health checks with your doctor (see column, p. 70) and consider taking HRT (see p. 74).

TAKE REGULAR EXERCISE

Investigators studying the relationship between bone density, prevention of bone fractures and exercise found that the amount of weight-bearing exercise, such as jogging, relates directly to increased bone mass. Women who take exercise twice a week have denser bones than those who take exercise once a week, who, in turn, have denser bones than those who never take exercise at all. It is never too late to improve your body. Bones can be strengthened to resist the effect of oestrogen depletion during the postmenopausal years.

If you are not physically active, ask your doctor about the best exercise programme for your level of fitness. Brisk walking will help to strengthen your bones. Try to exercise daily for 20–30 minutes, enough to moderately accelerate your pulse rate.

EAT A CALCIUM-RICH DIET

The most important dietary advice for the early prevention of osteoporosis is to eat calcium-rich foods. Calcium is lost from the body in sweat, urine and faeces, and maintenance of the correct amount is dependent on our dietary intake of calcium, combined with the presence of oestrogen and vitamin D. The bone deterioration that ends in osteoporosis begins a long time before the first fractures and the longer you wait to take action, the smaller your chances of recovery. In brief, to prevent your bones from becoming brittle, you need calcium for bone mass, vitamin D to absorb the calcium from your blood into your body and oestrogen to maintain the calcium inside your bones. For good food sources of vitamin D and calcium, see pp. 36 and 37.

BREAST CANCER

This is the most common type of cancer in women, and the leading cause of death in women who are aged between 35 and 50. In the UK, women have about a one in 11 chance of developing breast cancer.

Despite great advances in the technology used to treat breast cancer, the mortality rate has hardly changed this century. We do know, however, that the cure rate for breast cancer depends on the stage at which it is detected, and whether it has spread. The earlier any abnormality is discovered, the more likely it is to be cured.

Although there is no equivalent of the cervical smear test (see pp. 66–67), which detects precancerous changes in the cervix, an X-ray procedure called mammography exists (see p. 64), which is able to detect very small breast tumours that cannot be felt manually. However, sometimes early and curable breast tumours can be found by routine monthly examination, and all women should learn how to examine their breasts (see p. 63).

SYMPTOMS

A small tumour may be detected during a routine self-examination of the breasts. The most common site for a malignant breast tumour is on the upper and outer part of the breast, where a lump can usually be felt rather than seen. A tumour is rarely painful. Signs to look out for include nipple discharge, a newly inverted nipple, lumps or swellings in the breasts, armpits or along the collar bone and a puckered or dimpled appearance of the breast. (For Diagnosis, see column, p. 78)

MEDICAL TREATMENT

Radical treatments, for example partial or extended mastectomy, do not necessarily improve survival rates. Many surgeons now recommend lumpectomy combined with radiotherapy or anti-cancer drugs (chemotherapy).

Sometimes, before you undergo breast surgery, you may be asked to sign a form that will allow your surgeon to carry out treatment during an exploratory operation. Think carefully about this – you should always be an active participant in all decisions regarding your treatment. If there are signs that a tumour has spread to the lymph nodes in the armpit, you will need more extensive

RISK FACTORS

Certain dietary habits can put you in a higher risk group than average. There is a documented link between breast cancer and a high intake of animal protein, saturated animal fats and dairy products. Other risk factors are listed below.

Medium to high risk factors for breast cancer are:
• *Having a family history of breast cancer (especially close female relatives, for example, mother or sister).*

• *Early onset of menstruation and a late menopause.*

• *Being over the age of 40.*

• *Having children later than average.*

• *Being Caucasian.*

• *Being obese or having a diet high in animal dairy fat.*

Low risk factors for breast cancer are:
• *Having several children.*

• *Breast-feeding.*

• *Being short and thin.*

• *Late onset of menstruation and an early menopause.*

At one time, women taking oral contraceptives were thought to be at greater risk of breast cancer than women who did not take the pill. However, recent studies now suggest that there is no correlation.

DIAGNOSIS OF BREAST CANCER

The majority of doctors will refer a woman with a breast lump to a hospital so that further tests can be made.

If you have a cyst, the fluid will be removed and is usually discarded, as it does not normally aid diagnosis. A solid lump is examined using a procedure called needle biopsy. This is a virtually painless technique in which, under anaesthetic, a fine needle is inserted into the lump and some of the cells are drawn out. In 85 percent of cancerous tumours, malignant cells will be detected by a needle biopsy.

If a lump is small and not deep in the breast tissue, it may be removed with some surrounding tissue and examined in the laboratory. If cancer is discovered, blood tests, X-rays and bone scans will be carried out to help decide upon the appropriate treatment.

treatment in order to prevent any further spread. If your tumour is of a type that is sensitive to hormones, an anti-oestrogen drug may be prescribed.

Tamoxifen is a drug used in the treatment of certain types of breast cancer. It works by blocking the oestrogen hormone receptors in the breast cells and has fewer adverse effects than other anti-cancer drugs. Side-effects may include hot flushes, nausea, vomiting, swollen ankles and irregular vaginal bleeding. Women at high risk of developing breast cancer, for example with a family history of the disease, may be prescribed tamoxifen to help prevent any cancer from developing.

BREAST CANCER AND HRT

The use of HRT in women with breast cancer (past or present), as well as other female cancers, is controversial. Although many doctors regard breast and other cancers as a reason not to give HRT (see p. 58), some doctors will still prescribe it. Where appropriate, I have tried to reflect current medical thinking on HRT, but ultimately your doctor should decide your eligibility.

OUTLOOK

If a very small tumour is treated early, a complete cure is likely. All women who have had breast cancer will be asked to attend regular check-ups to detect any recurrence of the cancer or spread to the rest of the body. It is very important that regular breast self-examinations and yearly mammograms are carried out. Even if the cancer recurs, it can be controlled for many years with surgery, drugs and radiotherapy.

Comparative death rates from common cancers
Women become more susceptible to many types of cancer after the menopause. Breast cancer is the most prevalent cancer in women.

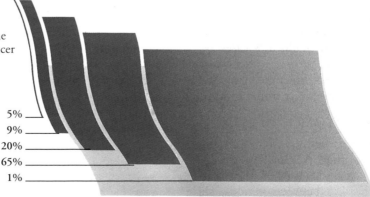

OVARIAN CANCER	5%
COLO-RECTAL CANCER	9%
BREAST CANCER	20%
OTHER CANCERS	65%
UTERINE CANCER	1%

THE UTERUS AND OVARIES

It's just good health management to have checks on all your reproductive organs at the time of the menopause when the hormones that keep them healthy start to wane.

OVARIAN CANCER

Malignant ovarian growths are most common after the age of 50; approximately 5,000 cases are diagnosed each year in the UK. Ovarian cancer is three times more common in women who have never had children, but less common in those who have taken the contraceptive pill. It may remain symptomless for some time and may be advanced by the time of diagnosis.

DIAGNOSIS

To determine whether a tumour is malignant or benign a laparoscopy will be carried out. This is an examination of the abdominal cavity through a fine fibre-optic viewing instrument. It is done through a tiny incision in the abdominal wall under general anaesthetic. If the tumour is very large, you may need an exploratory operation.

UTERINE CANCER

Unlike cervical cancer, which is most common in younger women (see Cervical Smear Test, pp. 66–67), uterine or endometrial cancer is most common in older women: three-quarters of all sufferers are over the age of 50, and very few are under 40. Between the ages of 55 and 65, the incidence of uterine cancer more than doubles. As the proportion of older women in the population increases, this upward trend is likely to continue. In the UK, there are nearly 3,500 new cases every year. Although cancer of the uterus is the third most common cancer of the female reproductive organs, it has a much better survival rate than cancer of the ovary.

SYMPTOMS

The earliest, most common sign of uterine cancer is abnormal vaginal bleeding, especially if you are postmenopausal. If you are still menstruating, any bleeding between periods, slight spotting, heavy and

TREATMENT OF OVARIAN CANCER

All tumours will be surgically removed, and microscopic examination of the cells will identify malignancy.

As much of the cancerous growth as possible will be removed, which may mean taking away part of the bowel, the Fallopian tube, the ovary and the uterus. Surgery is usually followed by radiotherapy and anti-cancer drugs.

OUTLOOK

If the growth is confined to the ovary, two-thirds of patients will probably survive for more than five years.

If the growth has spread, only one in five women will survive for more than five years. New techniques and drugs for detecting and treating ovarian cancer are improving survival rates. However, an annual ultrasound scan is the most important detection tool.

RISK FACTORS FOR UTERINE CANCER

Uterine cancer is more likely to occur among women who have never had children, and women of low fertility.

There is also thought to be an association between cancer of the uterus and oestrogen replacement therapy when it is taken without progestogen (see column, p. 47). However, nowadays HRT is prescribed in its combined form and this may actually protect women against uterine cancer.

Women who are obese (being overweight results in high blood levels of oestrogen), have a family history of uterine cancer, suffer from high blood pressure, diabetes, fibroids or disturbed menstrual patterns with long intervals between periods are all at a higher risk of developing uterine cancer.

TREATMENT OF UTERINE CANCER

A complete hysterectomy, with removal of the ovaries, Fallopian tubes and uterus, is the usual treatment.

In nearly all parts of the world this procedure, combined with radiotherapy in selected cases, before or after the operation, has vastly improved cure rates.

The overall cure rate is as high as 90 percent when the cancer is localized to the lining of the uterus and has not spread.

prolonged bleeding, or bleeding after intercourse are all symptoms that should be investigated. Advanced cancers may give rise to menstrual cramps, pelvic bloating and distension, with pressure in the lower abdomen. Symptoms affecting the bladder include frequent and urgent urination.

HYSTERECTOMY

This is the surgical removal of the uterus with or without other reproductive organs. In developed countries it is one of the most frequently performed operations, second only to episiotomy (surgical enlargement of the vagina during childbirth). You should always question your doctor's reasons for wanting to perform a hysterectomy.

WHY IS IT DONE?

• To remove cancer in the vagina, cervix, uterus, Fallopian tubes or ovaries.
• To treat severe and uncontrollable pelvic infection.
• To stop acute haemorrhage.
• When certain life-threatening conditions affect the organs lying close to the uterus, and it is technically impossible to deal with the primary problem without removing the uterus.
• To treat extensive and very painful endometriosis.
• To remove large or multiple fibroids.
• After injury to the pelvic musculature during childbirth, which is severe enough to interfere with bowel or bladder function.
• To treat heavy vaginal bleeding that doesn't respond to treatment and results in anaemia.

Although these conditions are all debilitating, there are some serious but poorly publicized side-effects associated with having a hysterectomy. Loss of sexual desire is quite common even if your ovaries are intact. A significant number of women experience a decline in their sexual desire after having their uterus removed, and taking HRT doesn't seem to help. Indeed, several studies show that HRT eliminates a dry vagina and pain on intercourse, but it does not influence sex drive.

There is also data from Scandinavia that suggests sexual activity is greater, and the incidence of painful intercourse lower, in women who do not have their cervix removed. Some women who had had a complete hysterectomy (involving the removal of the cervix) claimed there was a significant loss in their capacity for orgasm, and they experienced orgasm in intercourse less than one in four times. The presence of sensitive nerve endings in the cervix may play a crucial role in your post-operative ability to have an orgasm.

We know that the ovaries, even after they stop secreting oestrogen, continue to secrete androgens, and these hormones are very important in maintaining libido in women. Removing the ovaries during a hysterectomy denies a woman this sexual stimulant. However, if testosterone therapy is taken after the operation, some women notice that their sex drive returns to normal.

There are other important health reasons for retaining the ovaries. They are our main source of oestrogen, and we know that oestrogen deprivation results in an earlier onset of heart disease (see Hysterectomy and Ovarian Removal, p. 71) and osteoporosis (see p. 70).

All of these are indisputable reasons for discussing with your doctor exactly which reproductive organs will be removed. Do not make a decision without such prior discussion and ensure you have the power to make the final decision. Your partner will almost certainly support you in your decision. Make sure that he is involved in all discussions about treatment.

OUTLOOK

Many women are concerned that they will gain weight after a hysterectomy. Fortunately, this is a myth. A diet rich in fresh vegetables, fruit, fish and poultry will help you regain your strength and give you sufficient energy to start exercising and restore tone to flabby muscles.

Some women experience a psychological reaction after a hysterectomy. The following statistics have been compiled from various studies:
• Women who have their ovaries removed may blame the operation for hot flushes, lethargy and other menopausal symptoms.
• Women who have had hysterectomies are four times more likely to become depressed in the three years after surgery than other women.
• Depressed women who have had hysterectomies are likely to remain depressed for twice as long – on average two years – as women who have not.

WHY HAVE A HYSTERECTOMY?

A hysterectomy should be a comparatively rare operation. However, 30 percent of all women aged 50 and over in the United States have had hysterectomies, often when it was not absolutely necessary.

The removal of small fibroids, for instance, hardly warrants such a radical operation. Some doctors even advocate routine hysterectomy once childbearing is over. They argue that a hysterectomy forestalls the risk of cancers. Fortunately, this view is not widespread.

You should make certain that you and your partner are fully informed of the consequences of a hysterectomy, and have no reservations about such an irrevocable step. Remember, it is you who decides whether or not you wish to spend the rest of your life without your uterus.

Most medical conditions will respond to treatment without surgery if a doctor is positive and determined. I personally would never consider having a hysterectomy without obtaining a second opinion, regardless of persuasive arguments.

If your ovaries are removed as well as your uterus, you will experience menopausal symptoms after the operation. These can, and should, be alleviated by long-term HRT.

TREATMENT OF FIBROIDS

Small symptomless fibroids, which are often discovered during a routine pelvic examination, usually need no treatment except monitoring.

Surgery is required only for fibroids that cause symptoms such as pain or heavy bleeding. A hysterectomy (see pp. 80–82) may be considered if there are a large number of fibroids or if you are experiencing significant pain or pressure.

Myomectomy, which involves shelling the fibroid out of its capsule, saves the uterus and is an alternative.

If you are experiencing hot flushes and other menopausal symptoms, you should not necessarily be deterred from using HRT because you have fibroids. However, your doctor will want to carry out regular abdominal or internal examinations. Both the uterus and fibroids tend to shrink at the menopause, and the benefits of HRT in promoting good bones, a sense of well-being and improved sexual function need to be weighed against the inconvenience of symptoms due to fibroids.

- Women who have had hysterectomies are five times more likely to seek psychiatric help for the first time than women who have not.
- The majority of women who seek psychiatric help following a hysterectomy are those who were not suffering from a life-threatening condition. This suggests that if a woman believes her hysterectomy was performed unnecessarily, she may become depressed as a result.
- Women grow more dissatisfied with the effects of their hysterectomies as time passes.

FIBROIDS

These benign tumours grow slowly in or on the uterine wall, and their exact cause is unknown. Women who are below the age of 20 rarely suffer from fibroids, but they affect a fifth of women between the ages of 35 and 45, and a quarter of women over 80.

Progesterone production declines as women near the menopause, and the relatively unopposed oestrogen of the perimenopausal years may be responsible for the increasing number of fibroid tumours. Decreased levels of oestrogen after the menopause usually causes fibroids to shrink. When fibroids do increase rapidly in postmenopausal women, there are grounds for concern since these tumours have the greatest potential for becoming cancerous. Current dosages of HRT are not thought to be sufficiently high to affect postmenopausal fibroids one way or the other.

SYMPTOMS

Small fibroids may be symptomless. However, if a fibroid distorts the size or shape of the uterus, it may cause heavy or prolonged periods and anaemia. Large fibroids may press on the bladder, causing discomfort or frequent and urgent urination. Pressure on the bowel causes backache or constipation. Occasionally, a fibroid attached to the uterine wall becomes twisted on its stalk and can cause sudden pain in the lower abdomen.

DIAGNOSIS

Fibroids can cause the uterine wall to become lumpy and bumpy. If your doctor notices abdominal swelling he or she may recommend an ultrasound scan to confirm whether fibroids are present.

ATHEROSCLEROSIS

This is a disease of the arterial wall in which the inner layer thickens, causing narrowing of the channel, reduced blood flow and increased blood pressure (hypertension). The thickening is due to the development of raised patches called plaques inside the artery. These plaques consist of a fatty substance known as atheroma, and they tend to form in regions of turbulent blood flow, such as the junction of two arteries.

Atheroma worsens with age, causing irregularities in the smooth lining of the blood vessels and encouraging thrombus (abnormal blood clot) formation. Sometimes, a fragment of thrombus breaks off and forms an embolus, which travels in the bloodstream and blocks smaller blood vessels.

Atherosclerosis is a leading cause of death in the UK and atherosclerotic heart disease of the coronary arteries is the single most common cause of death. Strokes resulting from interference in the blood supply to the brain are the third most common cause of death (cancer is the second most common).

Atherosclerosis can also cause serious illness by impeding blood flow in other major arteries, such as those that supply the kidneys, legs and intestines. Before the menopause, women are protected from atherosclerosis by the body's production of oestrogen, so it tends to affect men and postmenopausal women. As most of the research on atherosclerosis and heart disease has been carried out on men, all statistics I have quoted relate to men, not women, unless otherwise stated.

SYMPTOMS

Until the damage to the arteries is severe enough to restrict blood flow, atherosclerosis is symptomless. When blood flow becomes impeded – generally after a number of years – you may experience angina (see p. 31), which is pain in the chest on exertion. Another symptom is intermittent claudication, which is leg pain brought on by walking and alleviated by rest. If blood flow is restricted in the arteries supplying the brain, you may experience temporary stroke symptoms, dizziness and fainting attacks. Kidney failure is also possible if the renal artery becomes narrowed.

RISK FACTORS

Obesity, smoking, high blood pressure, being menopausal and postmenopausal, lack of exercise, a high cholesterol level, poorly controlled diabetes and a family history of arterial disease all increase your chances of suffering from atherosclerosis.

A personality type known as type A, characterized by aggression and competitiveness, may also be a risk factor.

The incidence of atherosclerosis in women increases with age. In the 35–44 age group, coronary artery disease kills six times as many men as women. In the 55–70 age group, death due to atherosclerosis is nearly equal in men and women. This is due almost entirely to the decline of oestrogen levels during the menopause.

Women who develop heart disease after the menopause are more likely to have had excess body hair when they were younger (this occurs in women with high levels of testosterone). They should pay particular attention to the cardiovascular risk factors that are under their control, such as smoking, diet and stress levels. They should also discuss with their doctors the possibility of taking oestrogen in HRT to balance testosterone production.

SURGERY FOR ATHEROSCLEROSIS

People who don't respond to treatment, or who are likely to suffer complications, may need surgery.

A common surgical technique used to treat atherosclerosis is balloon angioplasty. This opens up narrowed blood vessels and restores blood flow. Coronary artery bypass surgery can restore blood flow to the heart, and a technique called endarterectomy can replace diseased blood vessels with woven plastic tubes.

DIAGNOSIS AND MEDICAL TREATMENT

Atherosclerosis can be diagnosed by angiography, a procedure in which a radio-opaque substance is injected into the blood vessels, enabling X-rays to show up the blood flow in an artery. Other techniques include Doppler ultrasound scanning (plethysmography), which produces a tracing of the pulse pattern.

Treating atherosclerosis with drugs is difficult, since by the time symptoms appear, the damage to the arteries has already been done. Although anticoagulant drugs can be used to stop further damage by preventing secondary clotting and embolus formation, they do not provide a cure. Vasodilator drugs will open up the arteries of the legs, and help to relieve symptoms.

PREVENTION

Lowering risk factors, especially in early adulthood and midlife, can help prevent atherosclerosis developing. If you smoke, you should try to give it up. You should have your blood pressure checked regularly and get treatment for high blood pressure. Lose any excess weight, keep your diet low in saturated fats, and if your cholesterol levels still remain high, you may need medication. Meticulous control of diabetes mellitus (see pp. 90–91) is important, and regular exercise is essential.

HRT may prevent coronary heart disease in that oestrogen has a beneficial effect on fat deposits in the blood, blood coagulation, blood glucose and insulin levels, and blood pressure. Women receiving HRT have half the risk of heart disease of non-users. This may be because they have higher levels of the healthy HDL cholesterol and lower levels of the dangerous LDL cholesterol that leads to hardening of the arteries.

Other new findings show that when oestrogen and progestogen are combined in HRT, blood glucose and insulin are lower and healthier in users than in non-users. High blood pressure should be treated before HRT is taken, but studies carried out in 1993 showed no rise in blood pressure in women taking HRT.

There is also a lower level of fibrinogen (a coagulation factor) in the blood of HRT users. This means that the blood is thinner and the likelihood of forming clots that might lead to a heart attack or a stroke is diminished.

UROGENITAL PROBLEMS

Hardly a woman beyond the menopause escapes some urinary symptoms because oestrogen is crucial in keeping the bladder and urethra healthy. Local oestrogen cream relieves many symptoms.

UROGENITAL AGEING

Oestrogen receptors are found in abundance in the genital organs, the lower urinary tract and the bladder, so the genital and the urinary organs can be treated as one system. When oestrogen is plentiful, the receptors keep this system healthy and resistant to infection. When hormone levels fall during the menopause, the receptors can no longer bind with oestrogen, and, as a result, are unable to keep organs strong and healthy. The urogenital system thins and becomes susceptible to infection.

SYMPTOMS

Signs of genital atrophy include a dry, itchy vagina and vulva, which causes pain during sex. These symptoms are often combined with the frequent, urgent desire to urinate and incontinence. This combination of symptoms is the most common reason for women over the age of 55 to visit a gynaecologist.

CYSTITIS

Oestrogen is so crucial to the health of the urinary tract that after the menopause the bladder is far more susceptible to bacterial infection. Cystitis is much more common in women than men anyway, because women have a shorter urethra (the tube leading from the bladder to the outside of the body). Nearly all infections that reach the bladder are due to bacteria entering the urethra from outside and then spreading upwards and inflaming the lining of the urethra and bladder. You should treat cystitis promptly because if it is allowed to recur it can become chronic, making it very difficult to eradicate.

SYMPTOMS

Only a woman who has suffered from cystitis knows how agonizing the following symptoms can be:
• The urgent need to pass urine frequently. You may start to pass urine involuntarily, and then find there

DIAGNOSIS AND TREATMENT

A bladder pressure reading will show if the bladder muscle contracts spontaneously causing urine to dribble away, leading to the symptoms of urgency and sometimes (but not always) incontinence.

A smear test (see pp. 66–67) will determine whether the vaginal lining has atrophied, with a loss of the protective acid vaginal secretions.

The first line of treatment should be oestrogen therapy. Research shows that oestrogen creams applied to the vagina diffuse through the urethra and the bladder and relieve symptoms in days. Oestrogen pessaries and rings are almost 100 percent effective. Oral and skin patch HRT (see p. 56) also eliminate symptoms.

CYSTITIS SELF-HELP

Right at the beginning of an attack, you should drink plenty of water or diluted fruit juice – cranberry juice is recommended.

Infection from the bacterium E. coli is the most common cause of cystitis. E. coli cannot multiply in alkaline urine, and you can make your urine alkaline by taking a teaspoonful of bicarbonate of soda in a glass of water. Drink this three times within five hours of the first twinge. Soluble aspirin and a hot-water bottle can help to relieve pain.

Each time you pass urine, pay attention to hygiene and wash your hands carefully before and afterwards. You should also wipe your perineum (the area between your vagina and anus) from front to back once with damp cotton wool. Soap and water can dry out the vagina and perineum and make you more prone to infection. When you dry yourself, pat gently – don't irritate the urethra by rubbing briskly.

If your cystitis is provoked by intercourse, it is probably best to refrain from sex until you are feeling more comfortable. Otherwise, reduce friction with a lubricating jelly and experiment to find the most comfortable sexual position. You should also wash carefully and pass urine after sex.

is very little urine to pass. This irritability of the bladder muscle is due to inflammation of the bladder lining, caused by the presence of bacteria. Even a few drops of urine can stimulate the bladder to contract.

• Severe pain and a burning sensation when you pass urine. This pain may occur when the flow begins and the bladder muscle starts to contract down on the inflamed lining, it may be during urination or it may be at the end, when the muscle squeezes the last few drops of urine out of the bladder.

• A dragging pain in the lower abdomen that may radiate up into the back. (Severe pain in the lower back could mean that you have a kidney infection and you should see your doctor immediately.)

• Blood in the urine can indicate severe inflammation of the bladder lining as well as a bladder tumour, so seek a medical opinion.

DIAGNOSIS AND MEDICAL TREATMENT

Your doctor will ask for a sample of your urine for analysis and for growing bacteria in a culture to see which particular bacterium is causing your symptoms. This will enable him or her to prescribe an antibiotic specifically to treat the bacterium.

Make an appointment to see your doctor as soon as possible, and take a specimen of urine in a clean receptacle with you. You will need a course of antibiotics and you should take the full course even though the symptoms may disappear within 36 hours. A minimum course for mild cystitis is three days, and in the case of a severe attack seven to ten days. With chronic infections, you may need to take antibiotics for three to six weeks.

Oestrogen cream, applied to the vagina by means of an applicator, will do a great deal to help prevent cystitis; oestrogen diffuses through the vaginal wall to reach the urethra where oestrogen receptors make the urethral lining healthy and resistant to infection.

PRURITIS VULVAE

Itching is a sign of oestrogen deficiency, and chronic, uncontrollable itching of the vaginal area is usually worst in hot weather or at night. Diabetes, vaginal yeast infections, such as thrush, and urinary tract infections, can all cause pruritis vulvae. However, it can be psychogenic in origin. Repeated scratching can become more and more pleasurable, even to the point of orgasm. Eventually, the sufferer will develop profound soreness and thickening of the skin in the vaginal area.

MEDICAL TREATMENT

Pruritis vulvae usually responds well to oestrogen cream. Your doctor can also prescribe an emollient cream that keeps the skin soft and well lubricated. You should apply these creams as directed. If there is excessive inflammation your doctor may give you a cream that contains hydrocortisone. If infection is suspected, he or she may give you a mild hydrocortisone cream containing an antibiotic. Oestrogen vaginal pessaries should also help.

If pruritis vulvae does not respond to treatment, your doctor can refer you to a dermatological specialist for further assessment of your condition.

INCONTINENCE

This occurs when the sphincter muscle at the base of your bladder becomes so weak (or the bladder muscle becomes overactive) that you have little or no control over the flow of urine. Although this condition is not life-threatening, it can be debilitating and embarrassing, and may make you housebound. Oestrogen helps to keep the sphincter muscle tight, and when oestrogen levels decline during the menopause, the muscle can become weak and flaccid, allowing leakage of urine.

The other probable causes of incontinence at or after the menopause are an irritable bladder, diabetes mellitus or local infections such as cystitis (see pp. 85–86). The three types of incontinence are as follows:
• Stress incontinence is when a small amount of urine leaks and dribbles away. It is caused by an increase in pressure inside the abdomen when you sneeze, cough, laugh or lift a heavy object.
• Urge incontinence occurs if you wait to urinate until you need to do so urgently. The bladder starts to contract involuntarily and empties itself. This type of incontinence is often triggered by a sudden change in position, such as standing up.
• Mixed pattern incontinence is a combination of both urge and stress incontinence, and may be the result of two faults in bladder function.

INCONTINENCE SELF-HELP

Mild incontinence is often due to weakened pelvic floor muscles, and you can improve your bladder control by doing Kegel exercises, also known as pelvic floor exercises.

These involve repeatedly contracting and relaxing the muscles of the urogenital tract (see Exercise and Sex, p. 26). If you are suffering from urge incontinence, self-help measures include emptying your bladder every two hours, and avoiding diuretic drinks such as coffee, tea and chocolate.

Aids for incontinence sufferers include waterproof bed sheets, incontinence pads, female urinals and waterproof pants. However, you should consult your doctor long before these become necessary. If you suffer from stress incontinence when you exercise, try emptying your bladder beforehand. Wearing a tampon during exercise can act as a splint to the urethra.

MEDICAL TREATMENT

Sometimes all you need to combat stress incontinence is oestrogen cream. Other forms of HRT will also help, and you should try consulting your doctor about them. Treatment may also include anticholinergic drugs, which are effective for an irritable bladder, an operation for stress incontinence and bladder retraining.

PROLAPSE

Prolapse, or "pelvic relaxation", occurs when the pelvic musculature is unable to support the pelvic organs and allows them to drop out of position. The affected organs include the uterus, bladder, rectum and urethra. The uterus is the most likely to prolapse. Because of advanced age, childbirth and a decline in oestrogen levels, the uterine muscles become weak and sag. The pull of gravity is a contributing factor. Prolapse is especially noticeable when abdominal pressure is increased by coughing or straining during a bowel movement.

FOUR TYPES OF PROLAPSE

Uterine Prolapse This type of prolapse is caused by a weakening of supporting pelvic ligaments and muscles. The uterus may descend from the pelvic cavity down into the vagina, causing irritation to the vagina, slight backache, and sometimes a sensation that your insides are going to fall out. The dropped cervix will also prevent deep penile penetration during intercourse.

Mild or first degree prolapse is when the uterus begins to descend into the vagina. Second and third degree prolapse are more severe. In second degree prolapse, the cervix begins to protrude from the vagina, and third degree prolapse is when the cervix and uterus protrude outside the vaginal opening. This condition is extremely uncomfortable and debilitating.

Prolapse is often the result of childbearing, especially if the pelvic floor muscle or the cervix was injured during delivery of a baby. Occasionally, the same conditions that have produced hernias in men, such as strenuous physical or athletic activity, may produce prolapses in women. Obesity and complaints such as constipation and chronic coughing all aggravate the condition because they increase the intra-abdominal pressure and cause the pelvic muscles to become weak and slack. Increased pressure can also lead to stress incontinence, in which you leak small amounts of urine when you cough, laugh, sneeze or lift heavy objects.

Urethrocele In this type of prolapse, the urethra bulges into the lower front wall of the vagina. Irritation of the urethral lining can lead to frequent urination.

Rectocele In this type of prolapse, the front wall of the rectum bulges into the rear wall of the vagina. Extreme discomfort is experienced when you have a bowel movement. In fact, it may be bearable only if a finger is inserted into the vagina to support the rear wall.

Cystocele The bladder bulges into the upper front wall of the vagina. This type of prolapse is nearly always accompanied by bladder problems, such as recurrent cystitis (see pp. 85–86). Sometimes the bladder sags below the level of the urethral outlet, which makes emptying the bladder extremely difficult. In such cases, it may be emptied by inserting a finger into the vagina and pushing up the sagging part.

MEDICAL TREATMENT

In the early stages of prolapse, HRT may help rebuild tissue structures that are inclined towards atrophy (thinning) because of low oestrogen levels. For older women, whose prolapse is not very severe, or where infirmity makes a general anaesthetic inadvisable, a ring or shelf pessary can be placed in the vagina where it supports the cervix and uterus. It should not be worn for very long periods because it may wear away the thin atrophied tissues by friction.

Surgery is needed for severe prolapse, when the cervix and uterus both protrude outside the vaginal opening. An operation is performed through the vagina and is tailored to the individual woman's problems. The anterior and posterior walls of the uterus can be repaired and the supports of the uterus shortened. If the uterus is severely prolapsed it can be removed. However, this is a major decision so discuss it thoroughly with your doctor or gynaecologist and seek a second opinion if necessary (see also Hysterectomy, pp. 80–82).

PROLAPSE SELF-HELP

These simple measures may help and are worth trying.

Wearing a girdle counteracts the dragging feeling that you may have and can relieve the discomfort to a certain extent.

Backache is one of the most common symptoms and it is very important not to stand for long periods, to maintain good posture and to rest with your feet up whenever you can.

You can protect yourself from prolapse by performing Kegel exercises (see Exercise and Sex, p. 26), avoiding over-strenuous activity, losing weight if you need to and giving up smoking, especially if you have a cough. Eat plenty of fibre, fruit and vegetables to keep your bowels regular and the stools soft (for ways to increase fibre in your diet, see pp. 37–38).

TREATING HYPOTHYROIDISM

Diagnosis is confirmed by tests that measure the level of thyroid hormones in the blood. Treatment consists of replacement therapy with the thyroid hormone thyroxine.

In most cases of hypothyroidism, hormone medication must be continued for life. However, if this treatment does not cure a goitre, surgery may be required.

SYMPTOMS OF DIABETES MELLITUS

Some women can suffer from a mild form of diabetes, which may be symptomless, although the condition can cause the following symptoms:

• *Damage to the back of the eye and blurred vision.*

• *Excessive thirst.*

• *Fatigue.*

• *Weight loss.*

• *Frequent urination.*

• *Itchiness of the vulva and vaginal infections.*

• *A tingling sensation in the hands and feet.*

OTHER HORMONAL CONDITIONS

All our hormone glands age as we get older and so the thyroid gland may underperform and a type of diabetes may emerge – both are easy to treat.

HYPOTHYROIDISM

The underproduction of thyroid hormones is caused by the body developing antibodies to its own thyroid gland, preventing the production of thyroid hormones. A condition called Hashimoto's thyroiditis is an example of this. More rarely, hypothyroidism may result from an operation to remove part of the thyroid gland, or from taking radioactive iodine as a treatment for a condition called hyperthyroidism (overactivity of the thyroid).

Hypothyroidism can occur at any age, but it is most common in elderly women. The condition affects one in 100 of the adult population.

SYMPTOMS

A deficiency of thyroid hormones can cause generalized tiredness and lethargy, muscle weakness, cramps, a slow heart rate, dry and flaky skin, hair loss, a deep and husky voice and weight gain.

A syndrome known as myxoedema may develop, in which the skin and other body tissues thicken. In some cases a goitre (an enlargement of the thyroid gland) develops, although not all goitres are caused by hypothyroidism. The severity of symptoms is dependent on the degree of thyroid deficiency. Mild deficiency may cause no symptoms, severe deficiency may produce the whole range of symptoms.

DIABETES MELLITUS

This is a deficiency of the hormone insulin. Sufferers whose bodies produce no insulin of their own and are dependent on insulin injections have type I diabetes. The type of diabetes that usually affects women over 40 is type II diabetes, in which insulin is still produced, but in insufficient quantities. This type of diabetes has a slow onset and may be discovered only during a routine medical examination.

Insulin, produced by the pancreas, controls the effective use of glucose in the body. Insufficient insulin makes the glucose level in your blood rise dramatically, and you start to excrete glucose in your urine instead of using it as energy, or storing it. The fact that you cannot utilize your most accessible form of energy has a detrimental effect on the body, and you may experience symptoms such as fatigue, weight loss, excessive thirst, the need to pass large amounts of urine, blurred vision and itchiness or redness of the vulva.

RISK FACTORS

Obesity is associated with diabetes. If you are overweight and have a high intake of carbohydrates, the amount of glucose in your blood will be high, and your pancreas may not be able to cope. Losing weight and changing your diet may be helpful. Other risk factors are heredity (a third of diabetics have a family history of the condition) and old age.

DIAGNOSIS

Your doctor will test your urine for glucose and a substance called ketones (a byproduct of fat breakdown). He or she may also take a sample of your blood after you have not eaten for a few hours. If both your urine and blood are found to contain significantly high levels of glucose and ketones, diabetes is likely.

MEDICAL TREATMENT

Serious cases of type II diabetes may need to be given hypoglycaemic drugs to lower blood glucose. Injections of insulin are not required since they are prescribed only for sufferers of diabetes mellitus type I.

The complications that can arise from severe diabetes mellitus include damage to the retina at the back of the eye (retinopathy), damage to nerve fibres (neuropathy), damage to the kidneys (nephropathy), atherosclerosis (see pp. 83–84), hypertension and gangrene.

Both diabetes and HRT alter the way that you metabolise carbohydrates, and for this reason HRT may be relatively contraindicated for diabetics. However, if your diabetes is stable, if you test your urine regularly, and if you liaise closely with your doctor, it may be safe, particularly in the very low dose skin patch form.

DIABETES MELLITUS SELF-HELP

It is important to monitor the amount of glucose you are ingesting. Too much glucose in the blood (hyperglycaemia) will exacerbate your diabetic symptoms, and too little (hypoglycaemia) will cause dizziness, weakness, confusion and finally unconsciousness.

You can monitor your glucose levels with a kit, which your doctor will give you, by dipping an impregnated strip into a sample of your urine and then comparing the colour change against a chart.

Your doctor will advise you about how to control diabetes with diet, but, as a rule, you should avoid all sugar. Eat small amounts of carbohydrates at regular intervals so that you do not have drastic fluctuations in glucose levels, and eat plenty of fibre (see pp. 37–38). In mild cases of diabetes that are due to obesity, simply cutting out sugar and reducing your weight will greatly improve your condition because your pancreas will be producing enough insulin to cope with your reduced body size.

ENJOYING LIFE BEYOND THE MENOPAUSE

As you grow older, you may go through a period of major reassessment. You may have a nagging feeling about something in your life you would like to change, but you may have deferred making changes because the time was never right. You may be dissatisfied with your job situation. You may feel that you don't spend enough time doing the things you want to do. You may want to make some changes in your relationship, or arrange some time away from your partner. If any of the above apply to you, confront your feelings and try to be honest with yourself. Talk over your thoughts with your partner, with friends, or perhaps even with a counsellor. If you let people know what you are looking for – whether it be a job or a new friendship – communicating your thoughts may open the door to new opportunities.

COMMIT YOURSELF TO ACTION

Once you've made up your mind about what you want to change and how to go about it, you must take the leap and commit yourself. This doesn't have to mean walking out of your job or filing for divorce, it just means taking a step in the right direction, whether it be registering with an employment agency or spending more leisure time away from your partner.

Try to avoid thinking of yourself as selfish – others close to you, such as your partner, can benefit from any changes that you decide to make. For instance, if you have spent most of your life at home bringing up a family, a new part-time job or a course could increase your sense of independence and make you feel more fulfilled, and this can have a positive effect on your relationship. You may have always wanted to follow a career and, as your husband approaches retirement, you could suggest swapping roles. Alternatively, you may be looking forward to a restful retirement.

Remember, you have already made many decisions and experienced many changes in your life and you're well equipped to cope with new experiences. Think of retirement as a period of self-renewal and it shouldn't be the crushing change that people often perceive it to be.

When asked what they miss most about working life, many people mention money and the social environment of work. However, there are very many advantages to retiring: you can follow your own body clock – eating, sleeping and studying when you feel like it; you no longer have to comply with authority; you have more time to spend on your family, friends and hobbies; and being out of the rat race can dramatically reduce your stress levels.

People usually start to prepare for retirement when they are in their 50s. You may start to reduce your job workload, seek financial advice or you may even decide to move to a smaller house. On a personal level, you may start to put more into your intimate relationships.

Whereas some people find retiring a natural transition, others, particularly women who have had fulfilling careers, may find it harder. We must prepare for this time since there may be little space for adjustment if we don't.

Retirement preparation is now a widely recognized need. Many firms, voluntary organizations and adult education centres give advice or run courses about financial planning, buying and dispersing personal property and assets, attending to health needs and organizing leisure time.

ORGANIZING YOUR TIME

Working fewer days in the week or less hours each day, taking longer holidays or working from home are just a few ways in which to make the move from paid work to retirement. If retirement could be less of a cut-off point and more of a transition, this might help to lessen its social stigma and improve emotional stability.

The loss of relationships at work following retirement, the departure of your children or even the death of your partner all mean that you may become more reliant on your friends and the younger members of your family. Friendships are important and likely to become more so as you grow older.

If you have time on your hands and feel at a loss, you are probably having problems making the emotional transition to retirement. Note times when your friends and relatives are free, and share your interests with them. Think up new projects and revive old hobbies. Sleep in late, meet a friend for lunch, read in the afternoon and put your feet up whenever you feel like it.

Useful Addresses

Age Concern
Astral House
1268 London Road
London SW16 4ER
Information line: 0800
009966
Website: www.ageconcern.
org.uk

*Provides information and
advice on coping with old age.*

**The Amarant Centre at the
Churchill Clinic**
80 Lambeth Road
London SE1 7PW
Helpline: 01293 413000

*Run by doctors from King's
College Hospital, London.*

Back Care
16 Elmtree Road
Teddington
Middlesex TW11 8ST
Tel: 020 8977 5474
Email: website@backcare.
org.uk
Website: backcare.org.uk

*Information on back problems
and their treatment.*

Breast Cancer Care
Kiln House
210 New Kings Road
London SW6 4NZ
Tel: 020 7384 2984
Helpline: 0808 800 6000
Email: info@breastcancercare.
org.uk
Website:
www.breastcancercare.
org.uk

*Offers advice, information and
counselling on all aspects of
breast cancer and its treatment.*

British Heart Foundation
14 Fitzhardinge Street
London W1H 4DH
Tel: 020 7935 0185
Email: internet@bhf.org.uk
Website: www.bhf.org.uk

*Offers advice on coronary
health and related matters.*

Family Planning Association
2–12 Pentonville Road
London N1 9FP
Tel: 020 7837 5432
Helpline: 0845 310 1334
Website: www.fpa.org.uk

*Provides written information on
sexual and reproductive health.*

**British Homeopathic
Association**
15 Clerkenwell Close
London EC1R 0AA
Tel: 020 7566 7800
Email: form on website
(below)
Website:
www.trusthomeopathy.org

*Information on homeopathic
medicine and registered
homeopaths.*

**Institute for Complementary
Medicine**
P.O. Box 194
London SE16 1QZ
Tel: 020 7237 5165
Email: icm@icmedicine.co.uk
Website:
www.icmedicine.co.uk

*Provides information on
methods of natural health care.*

Marie Stopes Clinics
153–157 Cleveland Street
London W1T 6QW
Tel: 020 7574 7400
Email: msi@stopes.org.uk
Website:
www.mariestopes.org.uk

*Information on sexual and
reproductive health.*

**National Institute of Medical
Herbalists**
56 Longbrook Street
Exeter EX4 6AH
Tel: 01392 426022
Email: nimh@ukexeter.
freeserve.co.uk
Website: www.nimh.org.uk

*Information on medical uses of
herbs and accredited herbalists.*

National Osteoporosis Society
Camerton
Bath BA2 0PJ
Tel: 01761 471771
Helpline: 01761 472721
Email: info@nos.org.uk
Website: www.nos.org.uk

*Advice on prevention and
treatment of osteoporosis.*

Open University
Walton Hall
Milton Keynes MK7 6AA
Tel: 01908 653231
Email: general-
enquiries@open.ac.uk
Website: www.open.ac.uk

Courses open to everyone.

Relate
Herbert Gray College
Little Church Street
Rugby Warwickshire CV21
3AP
Tel: 0845 456 1310
Email: enquiries@relate.org.uk
Website: www.relate.org.uk

*Counselling on all aspects of
relationships.*

Women's Health
52 Featherstone Street
London EC1Y 8RT
Tel: 0845 125 5254
Email:
womenshealth@pop3.poptel.
org.uk
Website:
womenshealthlondon.org.uk

*Information on women's health,
including the menopause.*

**Women's Nutritional
Advisory Service**
P.O. Box 268
Lewes, East Sussex BN7 7QN
Tel: 01273 487366
Email: wnas@wnas.org.uk
Website: www.wnas.org.uk

*Advice on diet to ease
menopausal problems.*

INDEX

ACKNOWLEDGMENTS

Dorling Kindersley would like to thank the following
for their contribution to this book:

PHOTOGRAPHY
Telegraph Colour Library for the title page.
All other photographs by Jules Selmes,
assisted by Steve Head.

ILLUSTRATIONS
Joanna Cameron, Tony Graham, Aziz Khan,
Joe Lawrence, Coral Mula, Howard Pemberton,
Sue Sharples

PAPER SCULPTOR
Clive Stevens

TP ASSISTANCE
n Shah

CONSULTANTS
Nicholas Siddle, MB, ChB, MRCOG; Neil D. Cox,
FBCO, FAAO; Sami Girling, MCSP, SRP, PGSDSP;
C.J. Hilton, FRCS; Diana J. Mansour, MRCOG

ADDITIONAL EDITORIAL AND
DESIGN ASSISTANCE
Nicky Adamson, Claire Cross,
David Summers, Ruth Tomkins

INDEX
Hilary Bird

TEXT FILM
The Brightside Partnership,
London